A Pompeian Herbal

Plant Portraits by Victoria I and Lillian Nicholson Meyer

Photographs by Stanley A. Jashemski and others

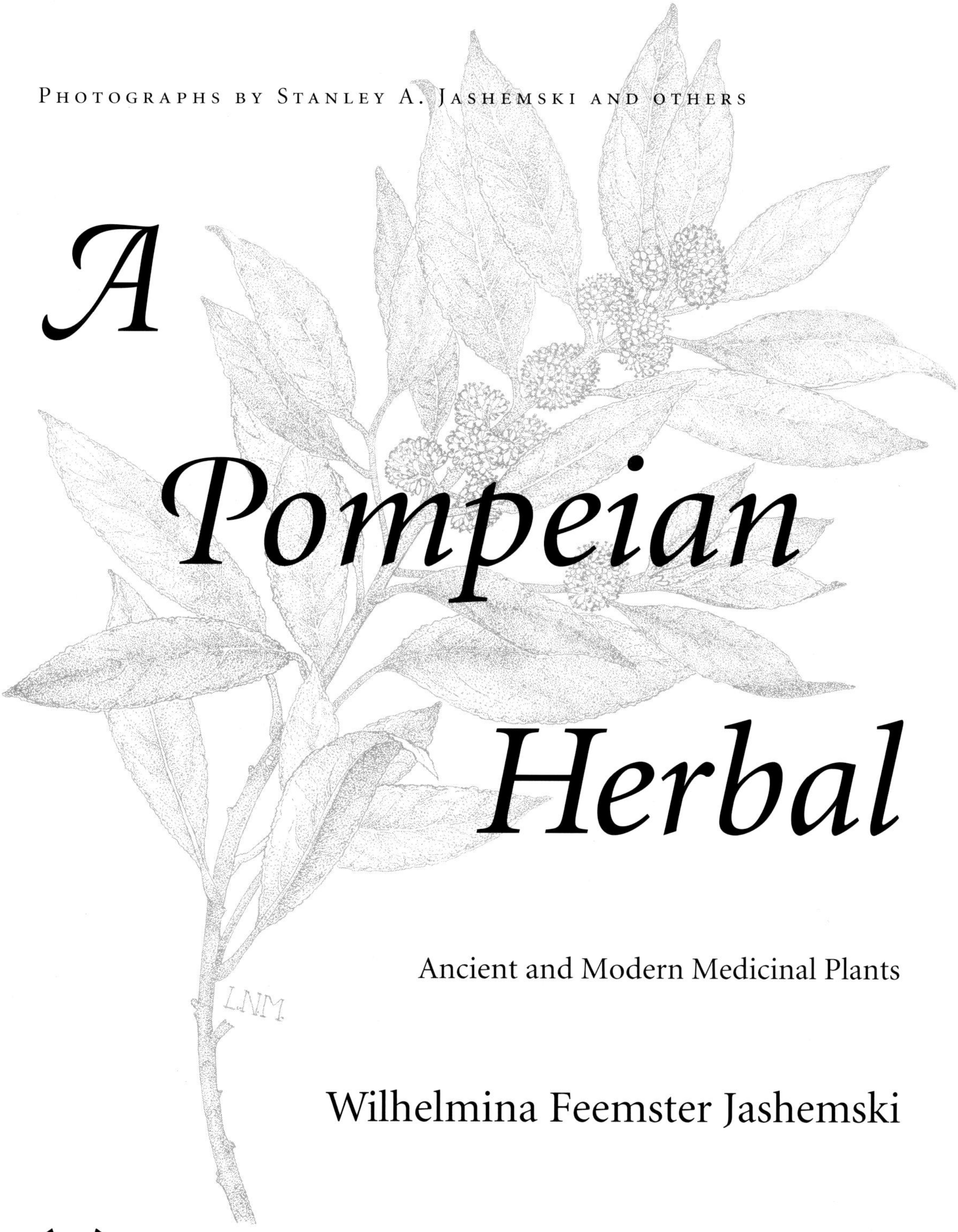

A Pompeian Herbal

Ancient and Modern Medicinal Plants

Wilhelmina Feemster Jashemski

University of Texas Press, Austin

Printed in China

First edition, 1999

⊗The paper used in this book meets the minimum requirements of ANSI/NISO Z39.48-1992 (R1997) (Permanence of Paper).

LIBRARY OF CONGRESS CATALOGING-IN-PUBLICATION DATA

Jashemski, Wilhelmina Mary Feemster, 1910–
A Pompeian herbal : ancient and modern medicinal plants / Wilhelmina Feemster Jashemski ; plant portraits by Victoria I and Lillian Nicholson Meyer ; photographs by Stanley A. Jashemski and others. — 1st ed.
p. cm.
Includes bibliographical references (p.) and index.
ISBN 0-292-74061-1 (acid-free paper)
ISBN 0-292-74060-3 (pbk. : acid-free paper)
1. Materia medica, Vegetable—Italy—Pompei.
2. Medicinal plants—Italy—Pompei. 3. Medicine, Greek and Roman. I. Title.
RS177.18 J37 1999
615′.321′09377—dc21 98-51226

Publication of this book has been generously assisted by grants from the National Endowment for the Humanities and the Gladys Krieble Delmas Foundation.

Contents

Abbreviations of Authors Cited or Quoted

Apicius	Apicius, *The Roman Cookery Book*
Celsus	Celsus, *De medicina*
CMG	*Corpus Medicorum Graecorum*
Columella	Columella, *De re rustica*
Dioscorides	Dioscorides, *De materia medica*
Galen, *De simpl. med. temp. ac fac.*	Galen, *De simplicium medicamentorum temperamentis ac facultatibus*
———, *in Hippoc.*	———, *Commentarii I in Hippocratis librum de humoribus*
Guarrera	Guarrera, *Il Patrimonio Etnobotonico del Lazio*
Martial	Martial, *Epigrams*
Ovid, *Met.*	Ovid, *Metamorphoses*
Pliny, *HN*	Pliny, *Historia naturalis*
Riddle, *Contraception and Abortion*	Riddle, *Contraception and Abortion from the Ancient World to the Renaissance*
———, *Dioscorides*	Riddle, *Dioscorides on Pharmacy and Medicine*
Scribonius Largus	Scribonius Largus, *Compositiones*
Soranus	Soranus, *Gynecology*
Theophrastus	Theophrastus, *Enquiry into Plants*
Tolkowsky	Tolkowsky, *Hesperides: A History of the Culture and Use of Citrus Fruits*

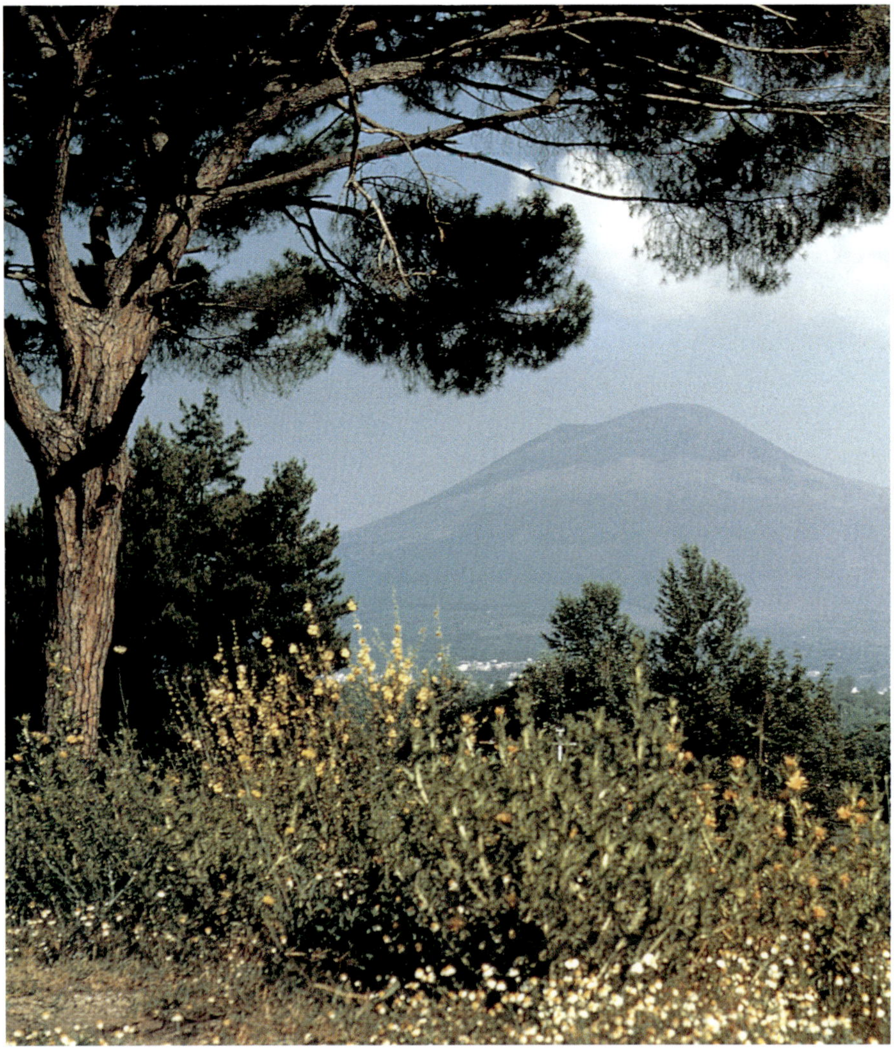

Medicinal plants growing at Pompeii in the shadow of Vesuvius

Preface

It is always a pleasure to express gratitude to those who have contributed to my work. Many people through the years have had an important part in the development of this book. It was first of all my workmen at Pompeii who introduced me to the herbs that they gathered to use as medicine. Then other workmen in the excavations, their friends and families, and also townspeople showed me the medicinal plants that they gathered, and explained their use. Dr. Pietro Soprano, Director of the Excavations at Pompeii, and later at Stabiae, gave me valuable information about medicinal plants in use at Pompeii and introduced me to neighbors living within the excavations who collected medicinal plants. It was he who directed a workman to get for me specimens of the miraculous "potato" (*Cyclamen hederifolium*) at Stabiae. The specimens that we collected of the plants being used for medicine are deposited in the U.S. National Arboretum herbarium in Washington, D.C.

In a book concerned with medicinal plants, the aid of botanists who know the flora of the area is indispensable. I have been fortunate in having the help and advice of four eminent botanists. For many years Dr. Frederick G. Meyer, Research Botanist in charge of the herbarium at the U.S. National Arboretum in Washington, D.C., now retired, has cooperated in my work on the gardens of Pompeii and the surrounding area. He has accompanied me on four trips to the Vesuvian sites and botanized the area, collecting specimens for the Arboretum herbarium, and he has documented many of the medicinal plants. His wife, Lillian Nicholson Meyer, a botanical artist, generously offered to make drawings of the specimens of the medicinal plants that I had collected.

Early in my research, I was privileged to meet the botanist Dr. Paolo M. Guarrera, now professor at the University "La Sapienza," in Rome, who was making a detailed study of medicinal plants used in Latium, the larger territory in which Rome is situated. From him I learned much. Professor Massimo Ricciardi of the Department of Arboriculture, Botany and Plant Pathology, University of Naples "Federico II" at Portici, who has closely collaborated with me in my work on Vesuvian gardens, has contributed greatly to this book. His interest in and knowledge of the medicinal plants used in the Pompeii area is considerable, and he generously gave me detailed information about plants he has used in treating his own family, in addition to other plants in the area used for medicine. He introduced me to Professor Matteo Giannatasio, a botanist at the University of Naples "Federico II," in Naples, who is also interested in medicinal plants. All four of these botanists have read my manuscript, and their corrections and suggestions have greatly improved it. Dr. Francis M. Hueber, chief paleobotanist at the Smithsonian Institution, Washington, D.C., has also aided my work, accompanying me on two trips to the Vesuvian sites. Four of his beautiful scanning electron microscope photographs appear in this book.

The untimely death of Lillian Nicholson Meyer, before she had been able to complete her handsome plant portraits for this book, made its publication very doubtful. I am much indebted to the gifted artist Victoria I, who generously offered to make the many additional drawings needed, thus making this book possible.

I have been fortunate in receiving many grants for my work, which I also acknowledge with gratitude, beginning with a grant from the American Philosophical Society. A Biomedical Services Support Grant aided my research on the medicinal plants used at Pompeii. Funds for my excavations in the Vesuvian sites were granted by the General Research Board of the University of Maryland, and in large part by the National Endowment for the Humanities, beginning with the award of a Senior Fellowship in 1968–1969 and generous research grants from 1972 to 1978. Dumbarton Oaks, Washington, D.C., also supported my excavations. The authorities at Pompeii and other Vesuvian sites generously furnished heavy equipment and additional workmen for my excavations.

It has been a pleasure to work with Jim Burr, the Humanities Editor of the University of Texas Press, and Carolyn Cates Wylie, the Managing Editor, who have so capably supervised the production of this Herbal. Marta Steele is the editor who did much to improve the book. We have been fortunate to have Heidi Haeuser as book designer.

Finally, my greatest debt, and one that never can be adequately expressed, is to my physicist husband, Stanley A. Jashemski, who played such a major role in my work. Taking leave without pay from his laboratory, he was every season an active member of our excavation team until his untimely death in 1982. His many contributions include the extensive photographic documentation of ancient Greek sites, and an even more extensive photographic documentation of the Vesuvian sites. His love of nature and of antiquity is reflected in his photographs that have found their way into the pages of this book.

A Pompeian Herbal

1 Introduction—Medicinal Plants: Then and Now

> Not even the woods and the wilder face of Nature are without medicines, for there is no place where the holy Mother of all things did not distribute remedies for the healing of mankind, so that even the very desert was made a drugstore. . . . Hence sprang the art of medicine. Such things alone had Nature decreed should be our remedies, provided everywhere, easy to discover and costing nothing—the things in fact that support our life. . . . But if remedies were to be sought in the kitchen-garden . . . none of the arts would become cheaper than medicine.
>
> —Pliny *Natural History* 24.1.1,4,5

I remember well the moment when I first became aware of the importance of medicinal herbs at Pompeii. It was an early summer morning in 1966 when we went into the *insula* (city block) across from the amphitheater to clear it of overgrowth before beginning our excavations. When my workmen spotted a patch of bright green weeds, they immediately rushed to dig them up and put them with their belongings, to take home at the end of the day (see Figs. 1, 2). I thought it very strange, and inquired why they did this. "For *fegato,*" they told me, "it is very good." I was to learn as I worked at Pompeii that liver (*fegato*) ailments were a common complaint, hence the importance of the medicine made from the herb that my workmen were gathering, the common weed known as mullein (*Verbascum sinuatum* L.).

As the days passed and my workmen continued to collect plants, I began to wonder if the plants they were collecting for medicine were the same ones the ancient Romans had used for cures. In my work I so often have been impressed

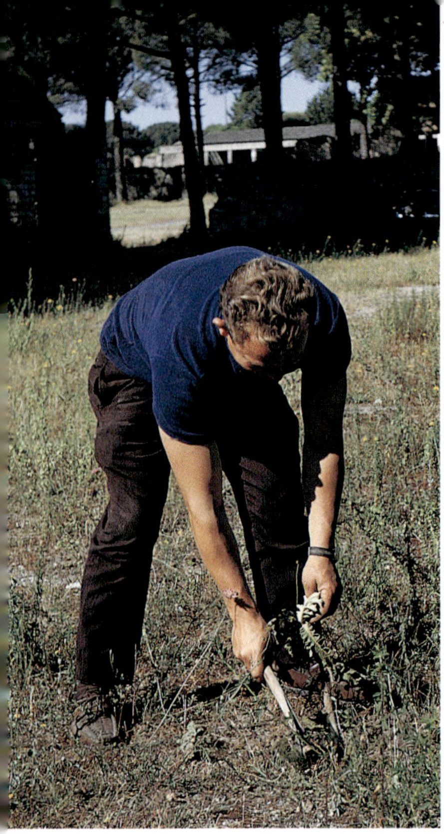

FIG. 1. Workman digging mullein for medicine

with the continuity of life in the shadow of Vesuvius. Frequently, when my workmen identified a new soil contour or other agricultural detail discovered in our excavations, I would ask them how they could be so certain. They would invariably reply, "Because we have always done it that way." When we uncovered a perfectly preserved hoe in our excavations, the happy worker who found it told me that he had a *zappa* at home that was an exact replica of the ancient one. The next morning he was at work early with the handle from his *zappa,* which fit the ancient hoe perfectly, ready to pose for a photo (see Fig. 3). Not far from the hoe, we found another ancient tool, an exact duplicate of the *martellina* that our workmen were using to clear weeds from the garden.

As I continued through the years to gather information about the medicinal plants used in modern Pompeii, I talked to many different people, some living in the country, some city dwellers, laypeople, and professionals (see Fig. 4). Again and again the same plants were mentioned—a limited but consistent list in which they placed great confidence. Among these were such common weeds as plantain (see Fig. 5) and purslane; there was also the lovely maidenhair fern, the fragrant alyssum, the ever-present bramble, or wild blackberry, bright blue larkspur, Apollo's laurel, even the English walnut, lettuce from the kitchen garden, and many others. It was exciting to discover the little white camomile with its yellow centers (see Fig. 6), chicory with its jewel-like blossoms of clearest blue, the beautiful red valerian (see Fig. 7), also "*verbascum* with the golden flowers," and the lacy St. John's wort (see Fig. 8).

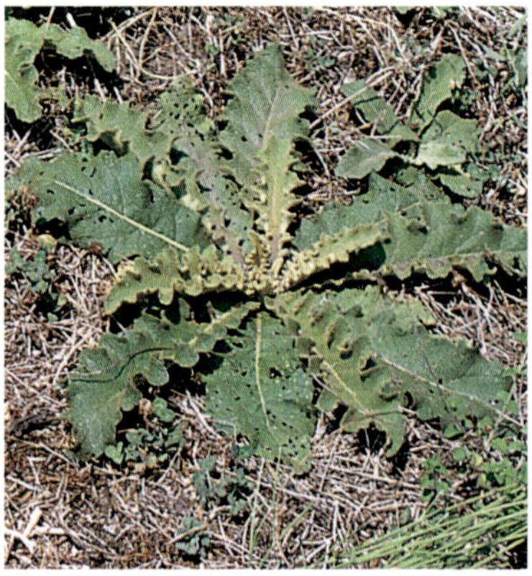

FIG. 2. Mullein plant with basal rosette of leaves

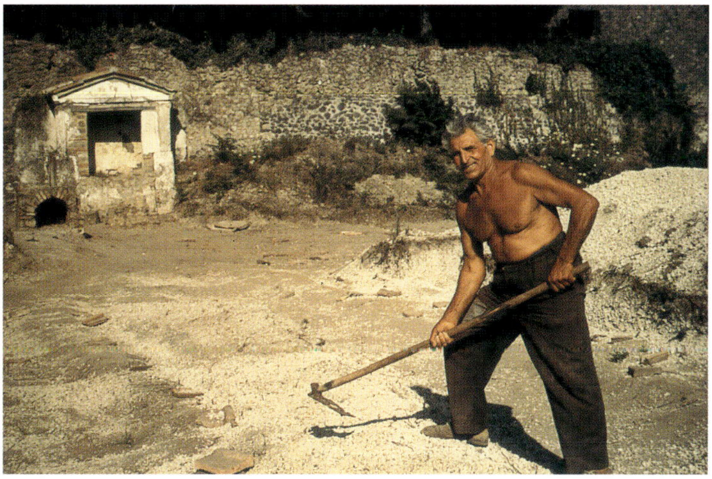

FIG. 3. Antonio and his *zappa*

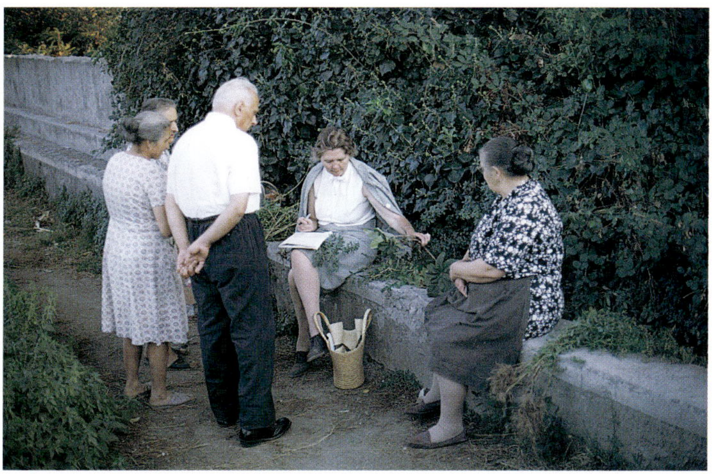

FIG. 4. Pompeians bringing plants to author, who records their medicinal uses and prepares specimens for deposit in the U.S. National Arboretum

We know that the ancient Greeks and Romans used medicinal plants extensively. Even the deities knew their virtues. The Roman poet Vergil recounts how, when the hero Aeneas suffered a deadly wound in battle and all attempts to heal him were in vain, his goddess mother, Venus, arrived on the scene with a stalk of dittany with downy leaves and purple flowers, which she had plucked on Crete's Mount Ida. After steeping the flower in river water, she gave the water to the aged Iapix, who washed the wound with it. Suddenly all pain left the body of Aeneas; the arrow which no one had been able to remove fell out unforced, and the eager

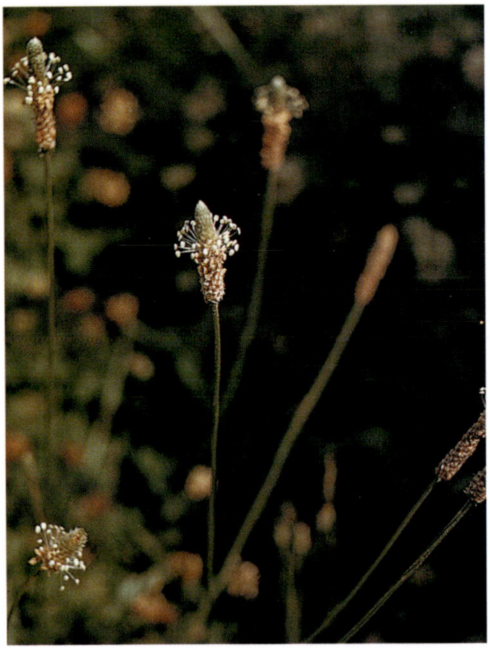

FIG. 5. Plantain inflorescence

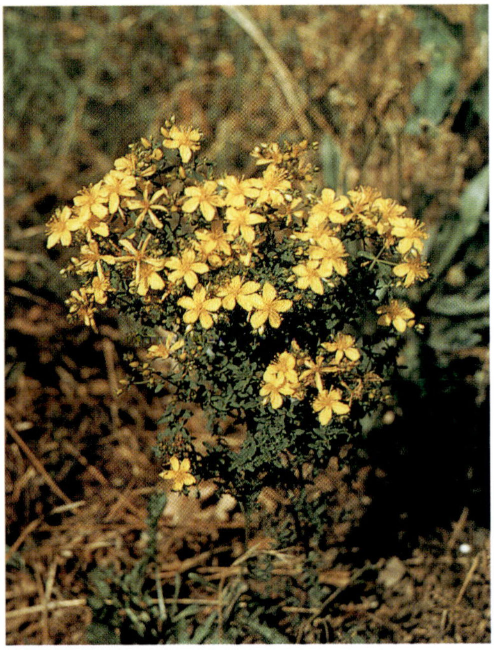

FIG. 8. St. John's wort

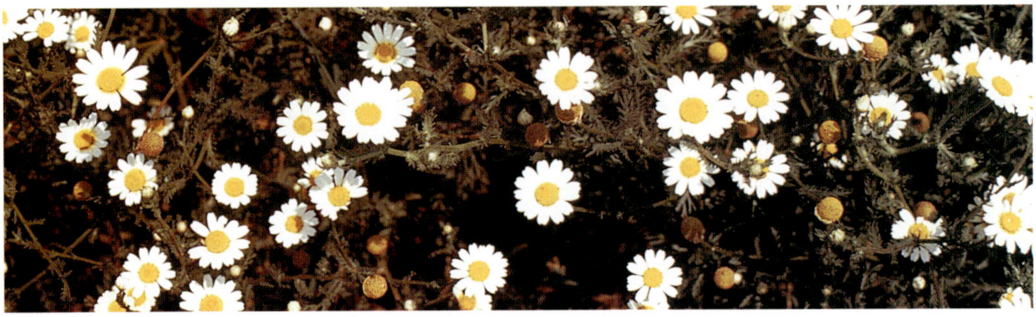

FIG. 6. Camomile

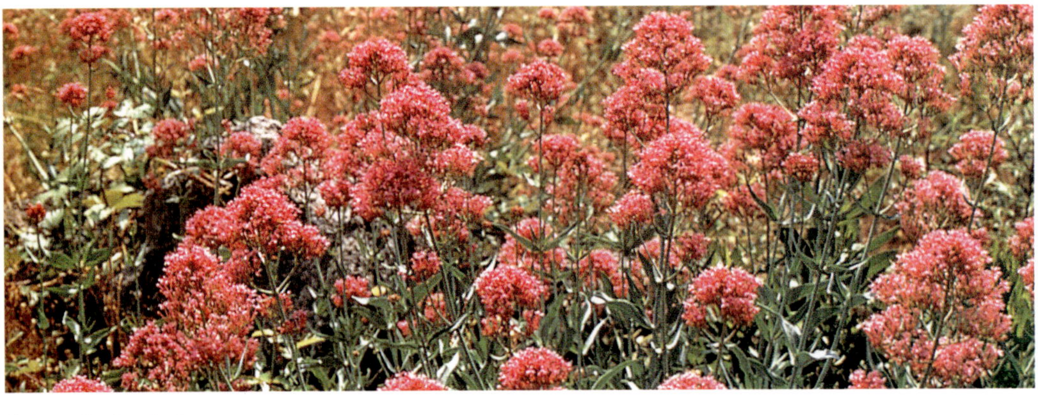

FIG. 7. Red valerian

Aeneas, with strength renewed, was ready to return to battle (*Aeneid* 12.411–431). Perhaps this episode reflects Vergil's early interest in medicine. He says that dittany was even used by wild goats, who cured themselves with it when struck by arrows. The Greek philosopher Theophrastus (ca. 370–288/5 B.C.), known as the "father of botany," in his *Enquiry into Plants* notes that dittany was peculiar to Crete, and that it was "said to be true, that, if goats eat it when they have been shot, it rids them of the arrow" (9.16.1). Pliny the Elder (A.D. 23/24–79) in his encyclopedic *Natural History,* often referred to as the *Encyclopaedia Britannica* of the Roman world, says that we learned from stags the value of dittany for extracting arrows from wounded flesh, for they ejected them by grazing on that herb (*HN* 8.97). A wall painting of Venus flying in with the healing dittany (*Origanum dictamnus* L.) for her son adorned the luxurious house of Siricus at Pompeii (located in Region VII, *insula* i, entrances 25 and 47) and is now in the Naples Museum (see Fig. 9).

Tradition is strong that Hippocrates (469–399 B.C.), the famed physician who lived on the Greek island of Cos, prescribed plant cures. Pliny the Elder frequently mentions the plants Hippocrates prescribed. On our first trip to Cos, many years ago, the local inhabitants proudly pointed out the aged plane tree near the harbor under which Hippocrates was believed to have sat as he wrote his prescriptions (see Fig. 10).

The present inhabitants of Cos, as elsewhere in the Greek world, continue to put great faith in the medicinal plants they gather. When I wrote to a Greek friend living on the island, inquiring about the plants she gathered, I experienced great difficulty attempting to explain that my interest was intellectual. She kept asking about the nature of my ailments, so that she could gather the appropriate plant and know whether leaf, flower, or root was needed. But she assured me of the efficacy of the remedies.

Hippocrates, the most famous of ancient doctors, was a contemporary of the philosopher Socrates and the historian Thucydides—three seminal thinkers of fifth-century Greece, who had great influence on subsequent thought. Just as Thucydides scientifically studied human political nature, Hippocrates studied our clinical nature and laid the foundations of medical science, for he developed practical medicine, fitting treatments to his diagnosis of each disease.

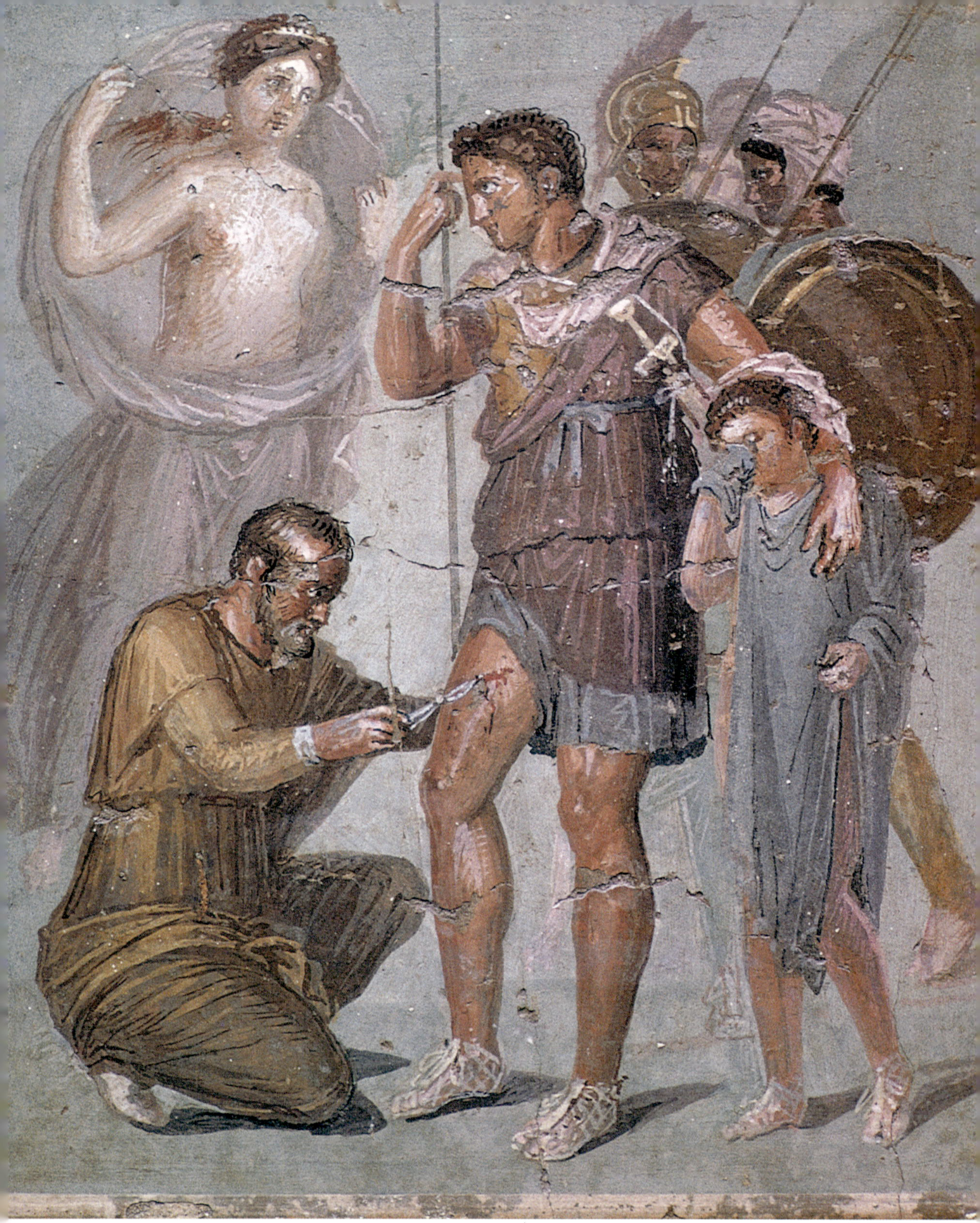

FIG. 9. Venus bringing healing dittany to Aeneas

The so-called Hippocratic Corpus, a collection of medical treatises, which contains important portions dating from the fifth and fourth centuries B.C., is not believed to include any actual writings of Hippocrates. But it may include teachings of the school of medicine which developed at Cos. From this corpus modern scholars have been able to put together a list of between four hundred and five hundred plants used as medicine, even though they are not discussed as a group.

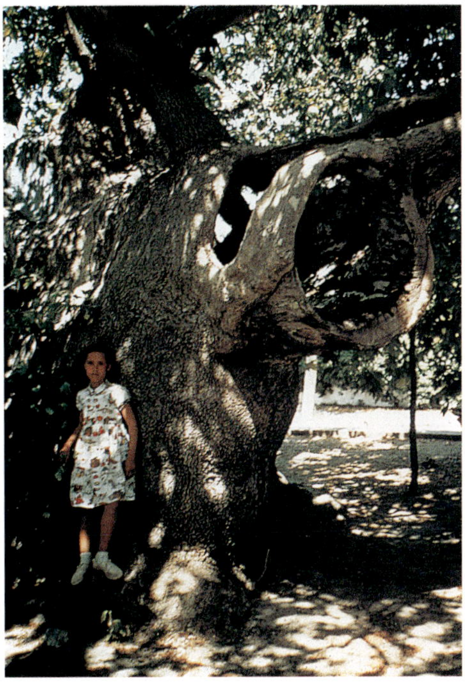

FIG. 10. Plane tree of Hippocrates at Cos

The first Greek writings to contain the names of many plants, and information about them, had a medical purpose. The physician Diocles of Carystus, a contemporary of Aristotle practicing in Athens about 350 B.C., was the first person to write a book (now lost) containing systematic descriptions of plants and the ailments they cured. Such a book became known as an herbal.

But it is from Theophrastus that we get our first detailed information about Greek plants (see Fig. 11). In his *Enquiry into Plants* he systematically applied the principle of classification to the vegetable world for the first time and described Greek plants. As a pupil and good friend of Aristotle, who had been the tutor of Alexander the Great, Theophrastus had access to the botanical observations gathered by the experts who accompanied Alexander on his campaigns. Theophrastus, however, says very little about the medicinal uses of plants, except in book 9, sections 9–12, which have the character of an herbal. Book 9 lacks the scientific character of the rest of the work and may have been added by another author after the death of Theophrastus.

The only Greek literary writer to pay substantial attention to plants was the first great pastoral poet, Theocritus, who lived a generation or two after Theophrastus had established the new science of botany in Athens. Woven carefully

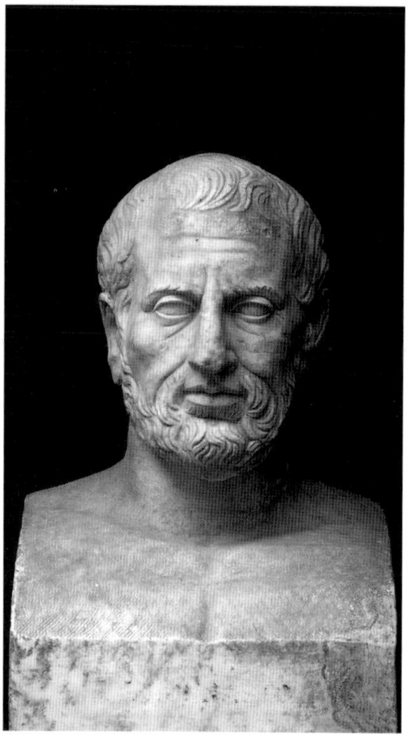

FIG. 11. Theophrastus

into the pastoral idylls of Theocritus are sensitive descriptions of many different trees, shrubs, flowers, grasses, and ferns, all in their correct habitat. In her study "Was Theocritus a Botanist?" Alice Lindsell argues that he had such training. Although a native of Syracuse, he lived much of his life in places outside of Sicily, including Cos, where he had friends and perhaps relatives. By the time of Theocritus, the famous school of medicine had been established at Cos. Tradition says that Theocritus studied medicine. This would imply the study of plants firsthand. Lindsell points out that Theocritus's descriptions could have been written only by someone who had carefully examined the plants, their flowers, and in some cases their roots.

The sanctuary of Asclepius at Cos today draws tourists from all over the world, instead of the sick, who thronged the shrine in antiquity, seeking healing. The healing god Asclepius had been venerated at Cos from earliest times. Originally the sanctuary had only an altar. Only after the death of Hippocrates in the mid-fourth century was the construction of the healing shrine begun. It is located on the ledge of a mountain about three kilometers beyond the ancient harbor town of Cos.

The completed sanctuary had four terraces, joined by monumental stairways (see Fig. 12). A wide stairway led from the lowest (fourth) level to a Doric propylaeum (temple-style vestibule), which gave entrance to the third terrace, the place of cure (see Fig. 13). This terrace was enclosed on three sides by a portico which gave access to the various rooms for the sick. From this terrace, a wide stairway led to the second terrace. At the top of the stairway, the ancient visitor faced the altar of Asclepius. On the right was the temple of this god, in which, the ancient writers tell us, many votive offerings, including votive statues of great beauty, were deposited. On the left was a temple built during the Roman imperial period. From

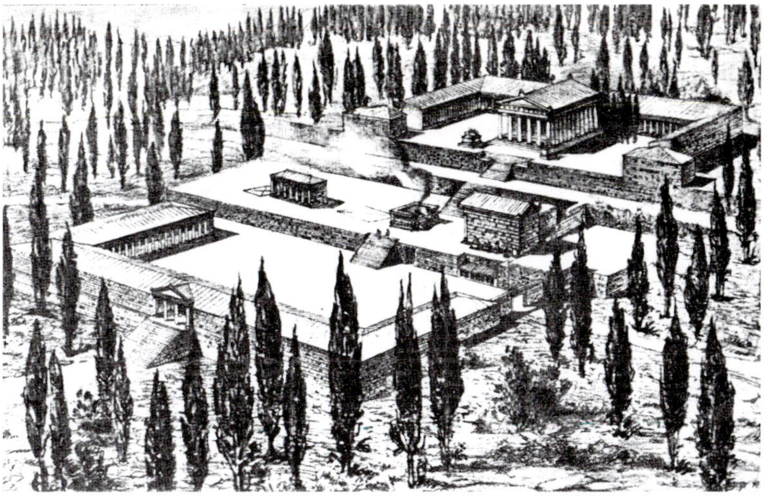

Fig. 12. Sanctuary of Asclepius at Cos: reconstruction

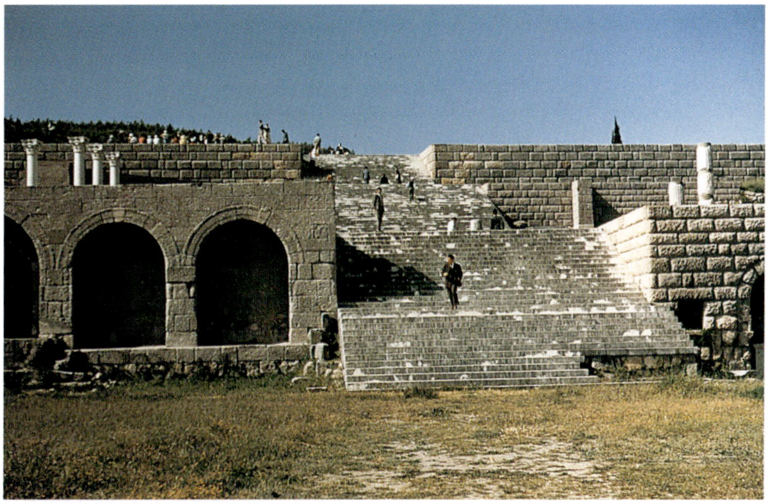

Fig. 13. Sanctuary of Asclepius at Cos: third terrace

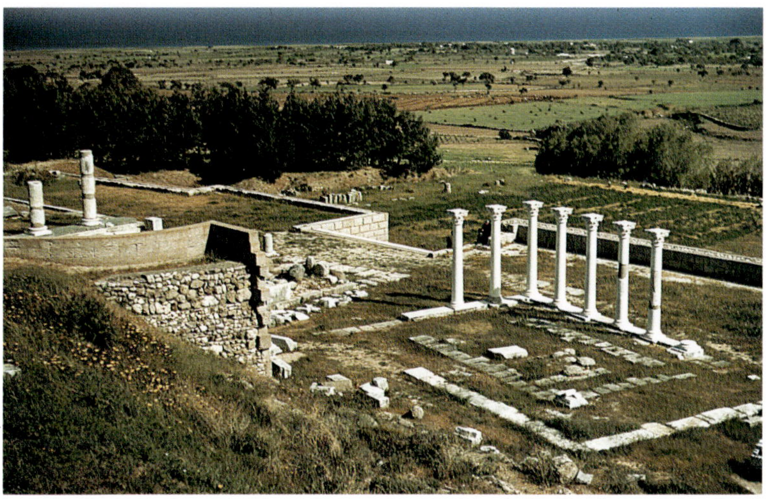

Fig. 14. Sanctuary of Asclepius at Cos: second terrace

this terrace we enjoyed the beautiful vista of the blue Aegean Sea (see Fig. 14). At the foot of the stairway leading to the top terrace are the scanty remains of a building in which the priests lived. A much larger temple of Asclepius crowned the top terrace, built when this terrace was constructed during the enlargement of the sanctuary in the second century B.C.

From Pliny the Elder we learn about a "very famous" herbal medicine used to counteract the poison of venomous animals, a medicine so important that the recipe was carved in verse upon a stone in the temple of Asclepius at Cos. He proudly gives the recipe, but not in verse:

> Take two denarii of wild thyme, and the same of opopanax [juice of all-heal] and of spignel respectively, one denarius of trefoil seed, of aniseed, fennel-seed, ami and parsley, six denarii respectively, and twelve denarii of vetch meal. These are ground and passed through a sieve, and then kneaded with the best wine obtainable into lozenges, each of one victoriatus [a coin, stamped with a figure of Victory, half a denarius in weight]. One of these is given at a time mixed with three cyathi [one-half cup] of wine. (*HN* 20.264)

He concludes with the information that King Antiochus the Great is said to have used this preparation as an antidote for the poison of all venomous creatures except the asp.

Any study of Roman medicinal plants relies heavily on Pliny the Elder's *Natural History.* At the time of his death, Pliny was the commander of the Roman fleet stationed at Misenum, across the Bay of Naples from Vesuvius. He lost his life when trying to rescue friends during the eruption of Vesuvius in A.D. 79. Sixteen of the thirty-seven books in his *Natural History* (books 12–27) are devoted to plants and their various uses. Books 20 to 27 are for the most part an herbal concerned with the medicinal uses of plants.

Another author of a very different type, and writing at about the same time as Pliny, is the herbalist-physician Dioscorides (fl. ca. A.D. 60–78). This skilled physician from Asia Minor includes more than five hundred plants in his herbal, which is written in Greek but better known by its Latin title, *De materia medica* (The materials of medicine).

Dioscorides tells us that he knew plants from studying them in the field, and not merely from books. But he studied carefully, drawing extensively on the works of predecessors. Of these, he writes most favorably of Crateuas, the rhizotomist (herb-gatherer or root-cutter) who served as the physician of Mithridates VI of Pontus (120–63 B.C.), who was also an herbalist. Crateuas, who has been called "the father of plant illustration," had painted likenesses of plants, under which he wrote their properties, in his herbal, which is lost. Such illustrations would have been of great help to the reader in identifying plants, in the days before plants had scientific names. Some scholars believe that the original herbal of Dioscorides had illustrations. If so, we can understand why so often Dioscorides gives no description of a plant, only its medicinal uses. The earliest extant illustrated herbal was made in Constantinople in 512 for Princess Juliana Anicia, and known as the Juliana Anicia Codex. The manuscript, known as the *Codex Vindobonensis Medicus Graecus,* is in the Austrian National Library in Vienna (see Fig. 15).

Pliny the Elder (see Fig. 18) was a busy lawyer active in affairs of state, not a botanist or physician, but he had a most inquiring mind and inexhaustible energy. He was essentially a compiler who drew heavily on the works of his predecessors. His nephew, Pliny the Younger (see Fig. 17), in answer to an inquiry from the historian Tacitus, described in a letter the way in which his uncle worked, finding time to write seven works filling 102 *libri,* or volumes. The *Natural History* was the last of his works and the only one that survives. Pliny the Younger's description is important to anyone evaluating the evidence in the *Natural History:*

> You may wonder how such a busy man was able to complete so many volumes, many of them involving detailed study; and wonder still more when you learn that up to a certain age he practiced at the bar, that he died at the age of fifty-five, and throughout the intervening years his time was much taken up with the important offices he held and his friendship with the Emperors. But he combined a penetrating intellect with amazing powers of concentration and the capacity to manage with the minimum of sleep.
>
> From the feast of Vulcan onwards he began to work by lamplight, not with any idea of making a propitious start but to give himself more time for study, and would rise half-way through the night; in winter it would often be at midnight or an hour later, and two at the latest. Admittedly he fell asleep very easily, and would often doze and wake up again during his work. Before daybreak

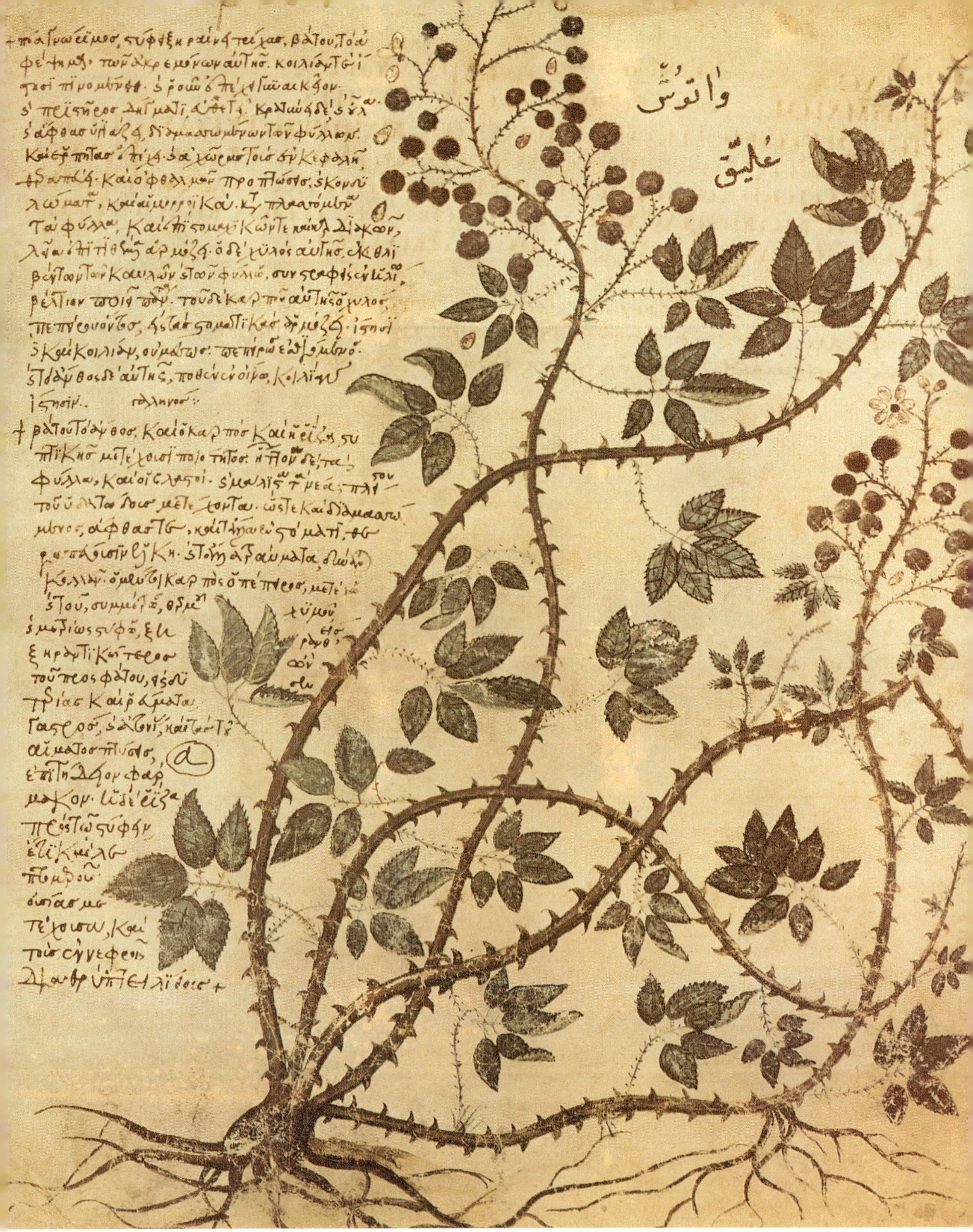

Fig. 15. Bramble, blackberry (*Codex Vindobonensis Medicus Graecus*, attributed to Dioscorides)

he would visit the Emperor Vespasian (who also made use of his nights) and then go to attend to his official duties. On returning home, he devoted any spare time to his work. After something to eat (his meals during the day were light and simple in the old-fashioned way), in summer when he was not too busy he would often lie in the sun, and a book was read aloud while he made notes and extracts. He made extracts of everything he read, and always said that there was no book so bad that some good could not be got out of it. After his rest in the sun he generally took a cold bath, and then ate something and had a short sleep; after which he worked till dinner time as if he had started on a new day. A book was read aloud during the meal and he took rapid notes. I remember that one of his friends told a reader to go back and repeat a word he had mispronounced. "Couldn't you understand him?" said my uncle. His friend admitted that he could. "Then why make him go back? Your interruption has lost us at least ten lines." To such lengths did he carry his passion for saving time. In summer he rose from dinner while it was still light, in winter as soon as darkness fell, as if some law compelled him.

This was his routine in the midst of his public duties and the bustle of the city. In the country, the only time he took from his work was for his bath, and by bath I mean his actual immersion, for while he was being rubbed down and dried he had a book read to him or dictated notes. When traveling he felt free from other responsibilities to give every minute to work; he kept a secretary at his side with book and notebook, and in winter saw that his hands were protected by long sleeves, so that even bitter weather should not rob him of a working hour. For the same reason, too, he used to be carried about Rome in a chair. I can remember how he scolded me for walking; according to him I need not have wasted those hours, for he thought any time wasted which was not devoted to work. It was this application which enabled him to finish all those volumes, and to leave me 160 notebooks of selected passages, written in a minute hand on both sides of the page, so that their number is really doubled. He used to say that when he was serving as procurator in Spain he could have sold these notebooks to Larcius Licinus for 400,000 sesterces, and there were far fewer of them then. (*Letters* 3.5.7–17)[1]

Pliny opens the first book of his *Natural History* with a covering letter to his friend Titus, son of the emperor Vespasian, to whom he dedicates the work. He

1. Reprinted by permission of the publishers and the Loeb Classical Library from *Pliny the Younger: Letters and Panegyricus, Volume I,* translated by Betty Radice (Cambridge, Mass.: Harvard University Press, 1969).

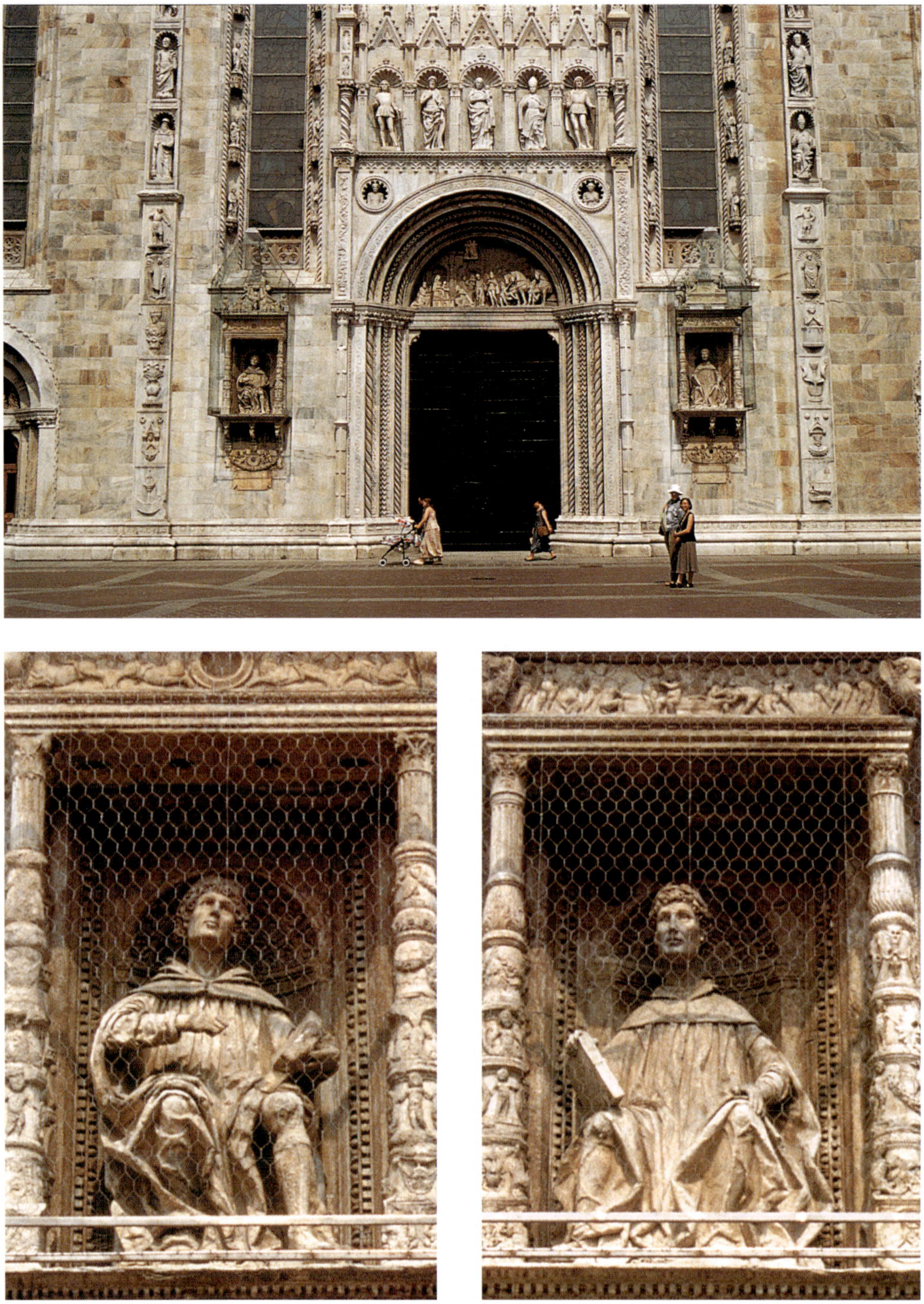

FIGS. 16–18. Como Cathedral (top). Pliny the Younger (left) and Pliny the Elder (right). The memory of the two Plinys, illustrious citizens of Como, has been venerated by their fellow townsmen ever since antiquity. Many years after their deaths their statues were carved on either side of the entrance of the 14th-century cathedral at Como, an unusual honor for non-Christians.

says that he has obtained his information from one hundred different authors, to which he added many of his own observations. The rest of Book 1 contains a table of contents of the remaining thirty-six books. At the end of the contents of each book, he appends a list of the authorities used, citing the works of both Greek and Roman writers. These include the Greek authors Theophrastus, Diocles of Carystus, and Crateuas. Among the Roman authors cited are Celsus, the poet Vergil, and the agricultural writers Cato, Varro, and Columella. Dioscorides is nowhere mentioned. But many passages in Pliny, as we shall see, are similar to some in Dioscorides. Pliny, however, is so scrupulous about listing his sources that we must conclude that both Dioscorides and Pliny borrowed extensively from the same sources. Although they were living at the same time, they did not know each other. Pliny had obviously read or heard Greek similar to that in Dioscorides' text, but Pliny's text is flawed due to his inferior understanding of the Greek. So there is no possibility that Dioscorides could have been copying Pliny.[2]

Indeed, Pliny is far more than a mere copyist and compiler. Professor Jerry Stannard, in his article "Pliny and Roman Botany," would go so far as to call him the "Father of the History of Botany." Pliny used illustrated Greek herbals, which could help in associating Greek plants with those of his native Italy. But more important, he also studied the actual plants. He tells us:

> I at least have enjoyed the good fortune to examine all but a very few plants through the devotion to science of Antonius Castor, the highest botanical authority of our time; I used to visit his special garden, in which he would rear a great number of specimens even when he had passed his hundredth year. (*HN* 25.9)

Stannard comments, "Were it not for this passage we should never know about the prototype of the modern physic garden."

A contemporary of Pliny is Celsus, whom Pliny quotes. Little is known of Celsus and, with the exception of a few fragments, little of his encyclopedic work on a variety of subjects remains, except his medical treatise, *De medicina.* This

2. W. H. S. Jones, Introduction to Pliny the Elder, *Natural History,* Loeb Classical Library (Cambridge, Mass., and London: Harvard University Press, 1951), vol. 6, p. xvii.

contains considerable information about plant cures. He begins this work praising medicinal plants:

> Just as agriculture promises nourishment to healthy bodies, so does the Art of Medicine promise health to the sick. Nowhere is this Art wanting, for the most uncivilized nations have had knowledge of herbs . . . for the aiding of wounds and diseases.

He continues by outlining briefly the history of medicine up to his time, giving an excellent summary of Greek medicine. His Latin is elegant, and the sound judgment with which he selected his material gives his *De medicina* great value.

The works of three ancient physicians also include information about plant cures, to be cited below. The Roman physician Scribonius Largus (ca. A.D. 1–50), a near contemporary of Pliny the Elder and Dioscorides, in his *Compositiones* (Prescriptions), his only surviving work, relies heavily on herbal remedies. But his lists of ailments cured by each prescription are far shorter than those of Pliny and Dioscorides. In A.D. 43 Scribonius accompanied the emperor Claudius on his campaign in Britain. Soranus of Ephesus, one of the greatest physicians of antiquity, practiced in Rome during the reigns of the emperors Trajan (A.D. 98–117) and Hadrian (A.D. 117–138) and was the author of almost twenty books on medicine. The *Gynecology* (Γυναικεῖα), his most important surviving work, lists medicinal plants used in treating women and young children. The physician Galen (A.D. 129?–199), whose writings survive in the largest number, had the greatest influence on subsequent generations. Although he was born about fifty years after the destruction of Pompeii, it is of interest to compare his prescriptions with earlier ones.

Archaeology has unearthed many material remains of the peoples of antiquity. But plants are very fragile and rarely survive. The extremely dry climate of Egypt has preserved some plant material in the ancient tombs. But such conditions are not found in Greek and Roman sites. It was therefore a rare and fortuitous discovery when several meters of carbonized hay were found in the Pompeii area, in a *villa rustica* at Oplontis (modern Torre Annunziata)—spectacular evidence for the flora of the area in antiquity.

The hay, brought to the villa from the site of its harvest in a vineyard, has been carefully studied by Professor Massimo Ricciardi and Dr. Giuseppa Grazia Aprile, who have thus far identified 128 taxonomic entities in the hay, adding 81 species, 37 genera, and one family to the list of 408 plants which, as P. A. Saccardo had previously shown, were probably known to the Romans in the first century A.D. Found in the hay are the carbonized blossoms, seeds, leaf and stem fragments, and pollen of many wild flowers and weeds (see Figs. 19–22), including some that are still used today as medicinal plants by the modern Pompeians. In 1983 a large amount of similar but less well preserved material was found stored in a room in a *villa rustica* at Terzigno, higher on the slopes of Vesuvius, but thus far it has yielded no new plants.

Pompeii and the other Vesuvian sites, because of the way in which they were preserved by the sudden and tragic eruption of Vesuvius, are a unique and precious source of information about ancient plants. In the many gardens, orchards, vineyards, and farmlands that I have excavated in the Vesuvian sites, we have found actual carbonized seeds, roots, fruits, and stems that enable us to identify the ancient plants. But such carbonized plant remains owe their survival to chance. They are preserved only in areas covered by pyroclastic flows, for such flows furnish sufficient heat to carbonize plant material. Unfortunately, most of the precious plant information preserved at Pompeii has been lost forever. Most of the city had been excavated before I began salvaging plant material for the first time. Our spectacular finds occurred in only a small part of the totally excavated area, often in sites where previous excavations had removed most of the lapilli that would have contained plant material. We still lack remains of many plants that we know were present during the Roman period.

Perfectly preserved planting patterns are another source of information. Invariably my workers recognized the patterns still followed in their own gardens. Pollen analysis is a further source of information. Contemporary refinements in the study of carbonized pollen have made possible the identification of many more ancient plants. But even information derived from pollen is limited. The area covered by volcanic ash does not provide ideal conditions for the preservation of pollen. Some of the pollen we found was badly damaged and could be identified only to family, not genus or species. Then too some pollens survive for a shorter time than others. Recently, a core taken at Lake Avernus by Professor

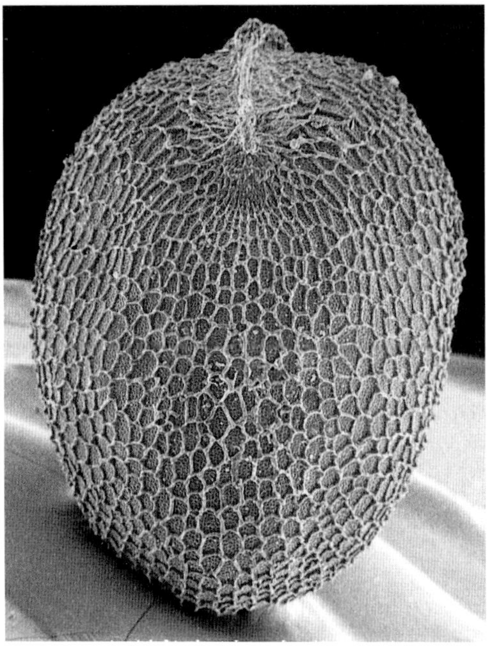

Fig. 19. Geranium seed (*Geranium rotundifolium*) SEM

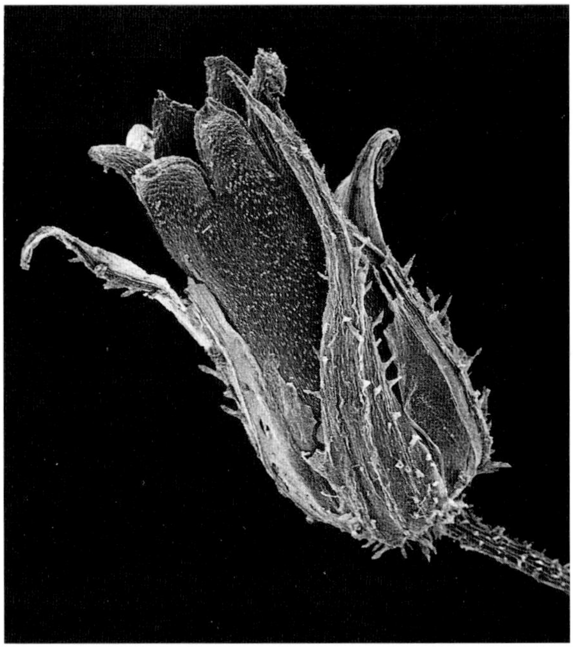

Fig. 20. Calyx enclosing ripe capsule, *Cerastium* sp. (pink family) SEM

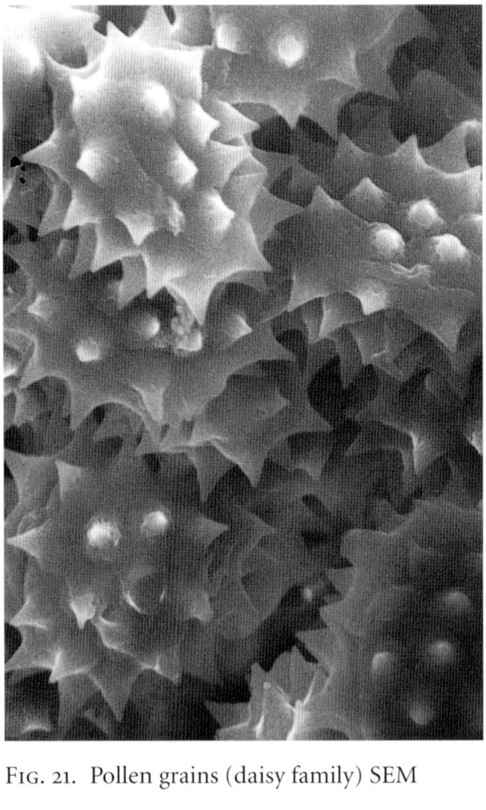

Fig. 21. Pollen grains (daisy family) SEM

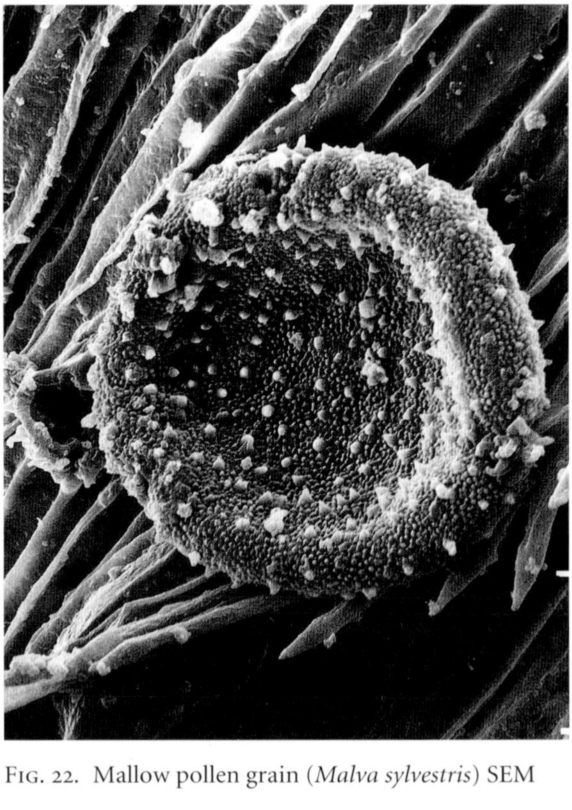

Fig. 22. Mallow pollen grain (*Malva sylvestris*) SEM

Eberhard Grüger and his colleagues has added tremendously to our knowledge of the flora of the area. For a detailed description of the flora of the ancient Vesuvian area, which includes a discussion of the various kinds of archaeological evidence, see the pertinent chapters written by specialists in the forthcoming book *The Natural History of Pompeii and the Other Vesuvian Sites,* edited by Dr. Meyer and myself.

Archaeological evidence is extremely important, for it is not always possible to know exactly what plant an ancient writer is referring to, especially if the writer mentions only the name of the plant and does not describe it. Some plants, which have had the same names since antiquity, can be identified without difficulty. For example, the ancient cyclamen (Greek κυκλάμινος, Latin *cyclaminos*), the ancient crocus (Greek κρόκος, Latin *crocus*), and the ancient chicory (Greek κιχόριον, Latin *cichorium*) are the same plants that we know by these names today. In some cases, however, unless the plant is described in some detail, the particular species cannot be determined. Identification becomes very difficult when the ancient authors refer to one plant by several names, perhaps using regional names, or use the same name for several very different plants. For example, the Romans gave the name violet (*viola*) to several entirely different plants. The name was used to refer to the sweet violet (*Viola odorata* L.), the stock, or gilliflower (*Matthiola incana* (L.) R. Br.) and perhaps the wallflower (*Erysimum cheiri* (L.) Cranz). Other violets mentioned by Pliny are unidentifiable.

It was not until the eighteenth century, when the Swedish botanist Carl Linnaeus devised a system of plant classification and consistently assigned to each known plant a Latin name called a binomial, or binary name (one for the genus, and one for the species), that greater stability in plant nomenclature was established.

As I gathered information about the medicinal plants used in the Pompeii area today, I discovered that almost all of them, according to the ancient authors, were used medicinally in antiquity. Today, however, a given plant is normally used for far fewer ailments, not as a panacea for a long list of complaints, including snakebite; but in most cases the present use was one valued in earlier days. At times it has been difficult to identify with certainty the exact species the ancient authors are describing. But various species of a given genus usually share common medicinal properties. Today medicinal uses of some plants vary in different parts of Italy, perhaps depending on local needs or traditions.

I have been able to get information about thirty-six plants collected for medicine in the Pompeii area, certainly a much, much smaller number than would have been used in antiquity, when plants were the principal source of medication. Animal and mineral products were used only to a very limited extent. Today the number of plants collected for medicine is decreasing rapidly. This does not mean, however, that plants are no longer used as medicine. With the increased industrialization of society, there is less time to collect and prepare plants for medicine. But they can be bought in stores that specialize in herbal medicine. I remember vividly the year I returned to Pompeii and discovered such a store directly across from the excavations. Fortunately, I began this study over thirty years ago, when it was still possible to preserve this valuable evidence, which represents such a direct continuity with the past.

In the text that follows, I have headed each entry with the scientific name, or names, given to the plant by Linnaeus or by a subsequent author, followed by the common name, or names, in English and in Italian. A short description of the plant is usually given, unless it is a very familiar plant. Any mythological associations with the plant are mentioned. The archaeological evidence for the presence of the plant in the Vesuvian area at the time of the eruption is noted. We have this kind of evidence for a majority of the plants described, with the exception of the eucalyptus, which is a newcomer. The remaining plants, believed to be indigenous to the area, would have been known to the ancient Pompeians, with the possible exception of the hollyhock and the alyssum. A description of the medicinal uses of the plant in the Pompeii area today follows, and finally the medicinal uses of the plant as reported by the ancient authors. (The translations of the ancient authors quoted are indicated in the bibliography.) The reader should be warned, however, of the potential danger of using any of the remedies described in this book. The dosage is important; some of the plants are poisonous even in small amounts and can cause miscarriage and various side effects. Facing each plant description is one of the beautiful plant portraits drawn by Lillian Nicholson Meyer or Victoria I.

As we explore the medicinal plants used at Pompeii today, discovering plants which the ancient inhabitants also knew and valued, we get still another glimpse into the lives of those people who lived so long ago, and with whom the present inhabitants feel a close kinship. There comes to mind an experience that happened during my early days at Pompeii, when one of my workmen proudly explained to me that one of his ancestors ran for office in ancient Pompeii. The proof: they had the same name, and it was painted on the walls, along the streets of the excavated city, on many an election notice in which the ancient candidate was asking people to vote for him!

II Medicinal Plants at Pompeii: Then and Now

1 *Adiantum capillus-veneris* L.

English, maiden-hair fern

Italian, *capelvenere*

Maiden-hair fern is a gracious perennial that grows wild around the Mediterranean in submountainous areas and the islands, in humid locations, near pools and on the walls of wells. Because of its beauty, it is a favorite in ornamental gardens. The Greek poet Theocritus (*Idyll* 13.42) mentions "fresh green maiden-hair fern" among the plants growing around the spring on the shore where young Hylas, the page of Hercules, went to fetch water. There he saw the nymphs dancing in the water, a sight forbidden to mortals. The nymphs, enamored of his beauty, pulled him into the pool. When Hercules tarried to look for him, the Argonauts continued their journey without him.

In the Pompeii area today, maiden-hair fern is used as a medicinal plant. I was told that five leaves taken as an infusion in a liter of water will cause an abortion. This use is also reported in the area near Rome (Guarrera, p. 27). In the Pompeii area maiden-hair fern is also used to prevent hair loss.

Maiden-hair fern was also used as a medicinal herb by the Greeks, who called it *adianton* (ἀδίαντον) (waterproof), a name retained by Linnaeus. Its use is mentioned in the Hippocratic Corpus. Theophrastus (7.14.1) lists only a few uses of the plant, one of which is that it prevents hair from falling out, as the modern Pompeians believe.

The Romans used the Greek name for this fern, calling it *adiantum*. Pliny's detailed description (*HN* 22.62–65) includes a long list of its many medicinal uses. It provokes menstruation. An interruption in the menstrual cycle could be due to pregnancy or to a variety of other causes. In ancient times there were no tests to determine pregnancy at an early stage. Any agent that provokes menstruation (an emmenagogue) in fact could cause an early-stage abortion. Pliny says that this fern is called by some "lovely hair or thick hair," because it dyes the hair when it is mixed with wine, celery seed, and oil and makes the hair grow curly and thick. He prescribes it to keep hair from falling out, as do the modern Pompeians. Dioscorides (4.136) lists much the same uses of *adiantum* (ἀδίαντον). He, too, says that this fern provokes menstruation and prevents hair from falling out. This fern was also known as the hair of Venus (*capillus veneris*) (according to an anonymous herbal of the fourth century A.D., attributed to Apuleius Platonicus), a name which Linnaeus incorporated into its scientific name.

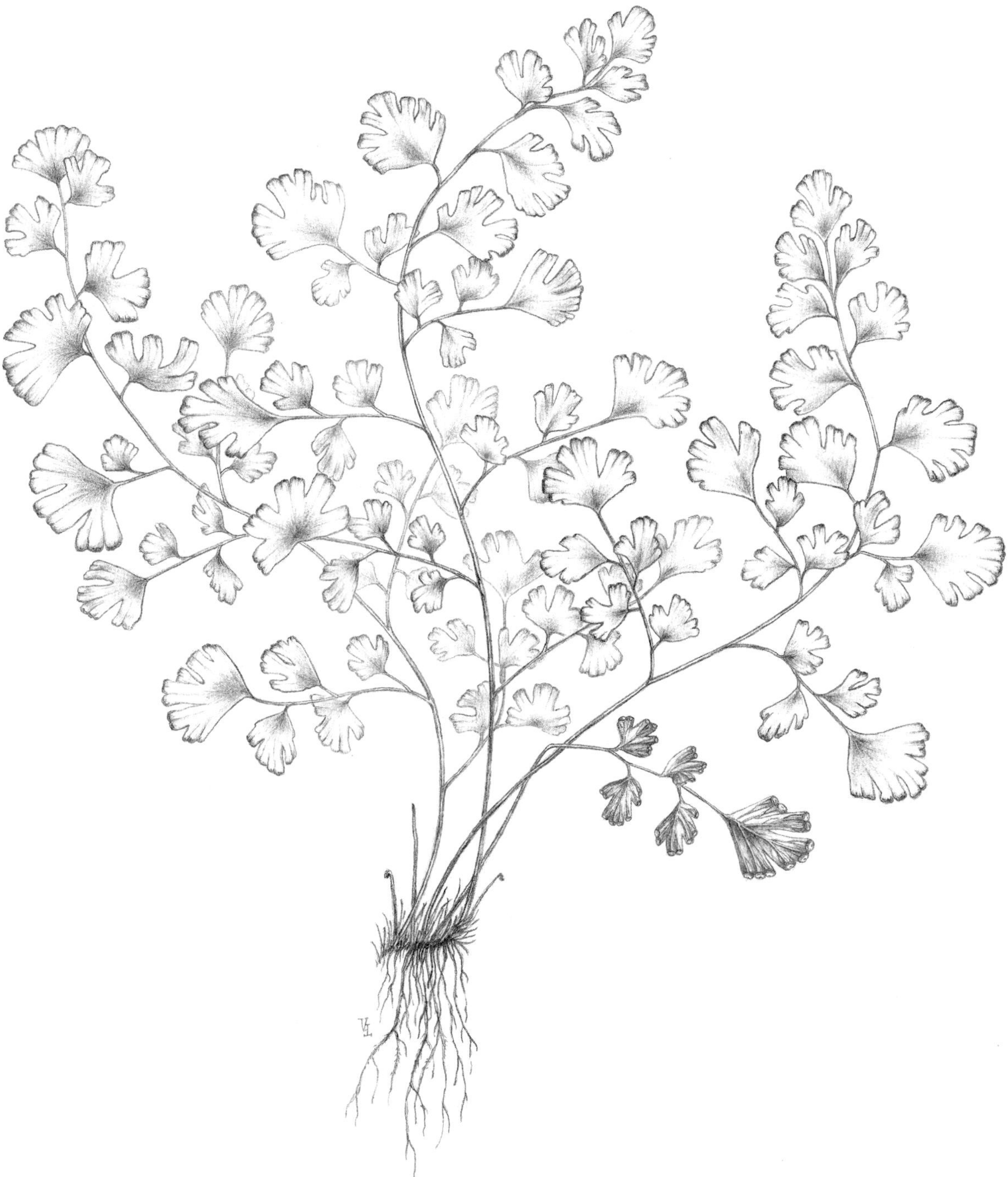

2 *Alcea rosea* L.

(*Althaea rosea* (L.) Cav.)

English, hollyhock

Italian, *malvone, malvarosa*

In Pompeii, flowers of the hollyhock, long a favorite in the old-fashioned cottage flower garden, are boiled in water to make a cough medicine, in which the Pompeians have great confidence. Hollyhock flowers and apples boiled together are given to *bambini* for stomach ailments.

Scholars are not agreed as to the origin of the hollyhock. Nor do they know how early it was grown in Italy. Some believe that Columella in his treatise *On Agriculture* (10.247) is referring to the hollyhock when he speaks of the "mallow whose bended head follows the sun."

According to Gunther, Dioscorides is discussing both the hollyhock (*Alcea rosea*) and the common mallow (*Malva sylvestris*) (see below, no. 24), in the passage (2.144) in which he speaks of both a cultivated (μαλάχη κηπαῖα) and a wild (μαλάχη ἄγρια) plant.

Riddle (*Dioscorides,* p. 65) also translates μαλάχη κηπαῖα as "hollyhock." He points out that Dioscorides' discussion of the hollyhock reveals how refined in description he could be: hollyhock is "bad for the upper tract, good for the lower, and profitable for the intestines and bladder."

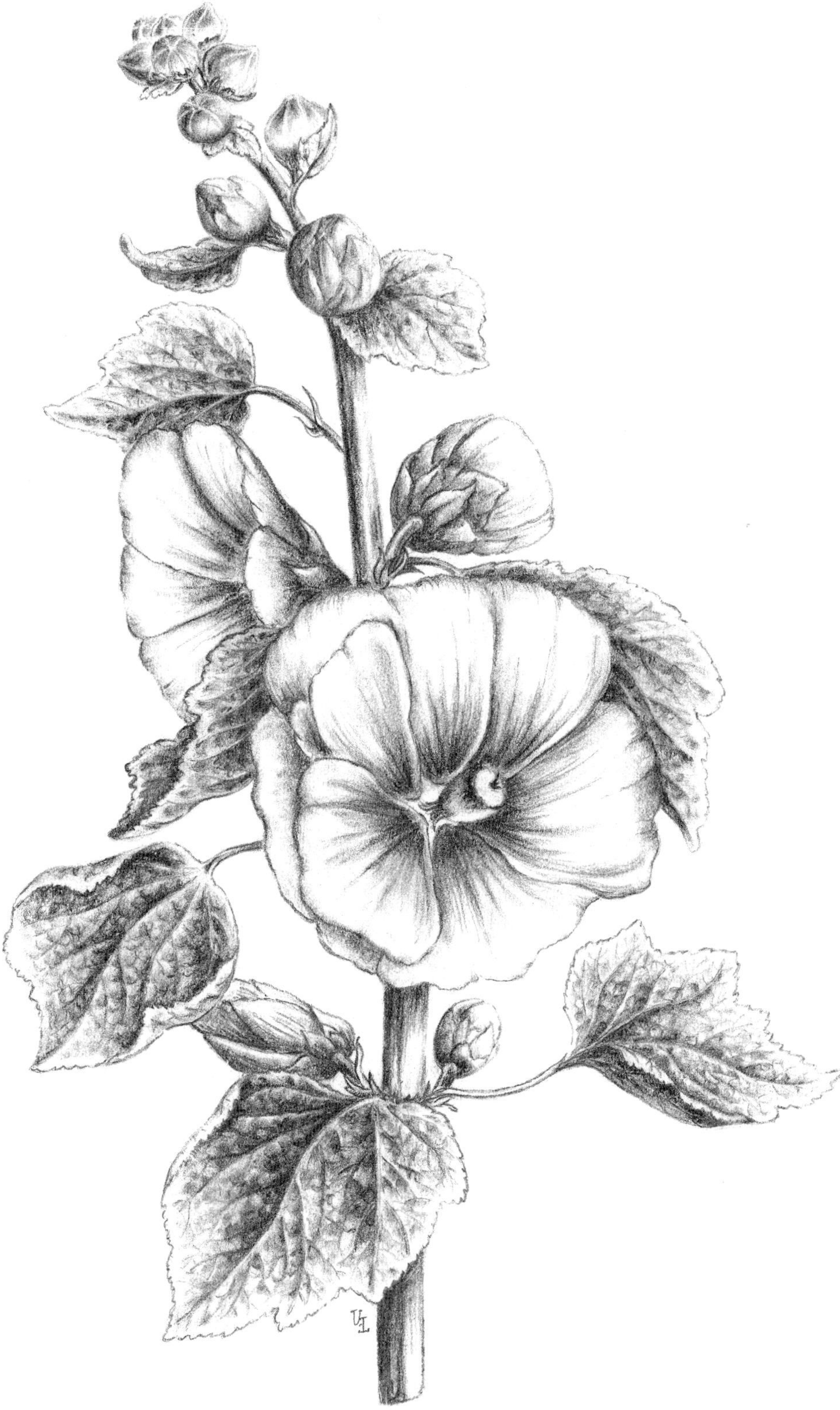

3 *Artemisia absinthium* L.

English, common wormwood

Italian, *assenzio*

This herbaceous perennial with racemes of small, pale yellow flowers is known at Pompeii by its Neapolitan name, *rescenzo.* It has very soft silky leaves, green on the upper, white on the lower surface and grows thirty to one hundred centimeters tall. Wormwood was a common weed in ancient Pompeii, as is shown by the wormwood pollen identified in the ancient gardens and nearby farmland in the *villa rustica,* in the *località villa Regina,* at Boscoreale that I excavated.

The women living within the excavations recommended boiling wormwood in water and using the infusion for colitis. A priest at Pompeii assured me that it was effective for diabetes; two branches about thirty centimeters long are boiled in a half-liter of water for a few minutes, and when cool a glassful is drunk once a day. The nuns at Pompeii had prescribed this remedy for him. It is also used to flavor vermouth.

Theophrastus (7.9.5) says the leaves and stems of wormwood (ἀψίνθιον) are bitter but wholesome. Columella (12.35) gives a recipe for making wormwood-flavored wine using Pontic wormwood, which the Romans considered choice and less bitter than the Italian variety. Absinthe has long been used as the base of many liquors, but the plant is poisonous and its continued use can cause irreversible degeneration of the brain; thus many countries now forbid its use.

According to Pliny (*HN* 27.45–53) the Romans used wormwood (*absinthium*) most often by infusing it in water. It was also used by the ancient Romans for colitis, as in modern Pompeii, to soothe the bowels, curing them when they are in pain, and for many other ailments; they also used it as an emmenagogue (*HN* 26.151). Dioscorides (3.26) lists among its wide variety of applications its usefulness as an emmenagogue. Used with myrrh or the juice of rue, it is an emmenagogue and abortifacient (1.77). Scribonius (227) uses *absinthium* in a prescription for hemorrhoids.

Soranus (1.65) lists it as one of the plants used in making a gentle abortive vaginal suppository. It is known today that wormwood causes abortions and is a contraceptive. Celsus prescribes wormwood for a variety of ailments: as a diuretic (2.31), for jaundice (3.24.2), and as a remedy in treating children with worms (4.24.2). Santonin, derived from the dried flower heads of a species of artemisia, is still used today to treat intestinal worms.

Wormwood had been employed from earliest times in the sacred rites of Rome (Pliny, *HN* 27.45). At the Latin festival, a serious ancient festival that had become a symbol of Rome's worldwide empire, the winner of the four-horse chariot race was given a wormwood drink, for, as Pliny says, it was believed that health was a very fine gift to give.

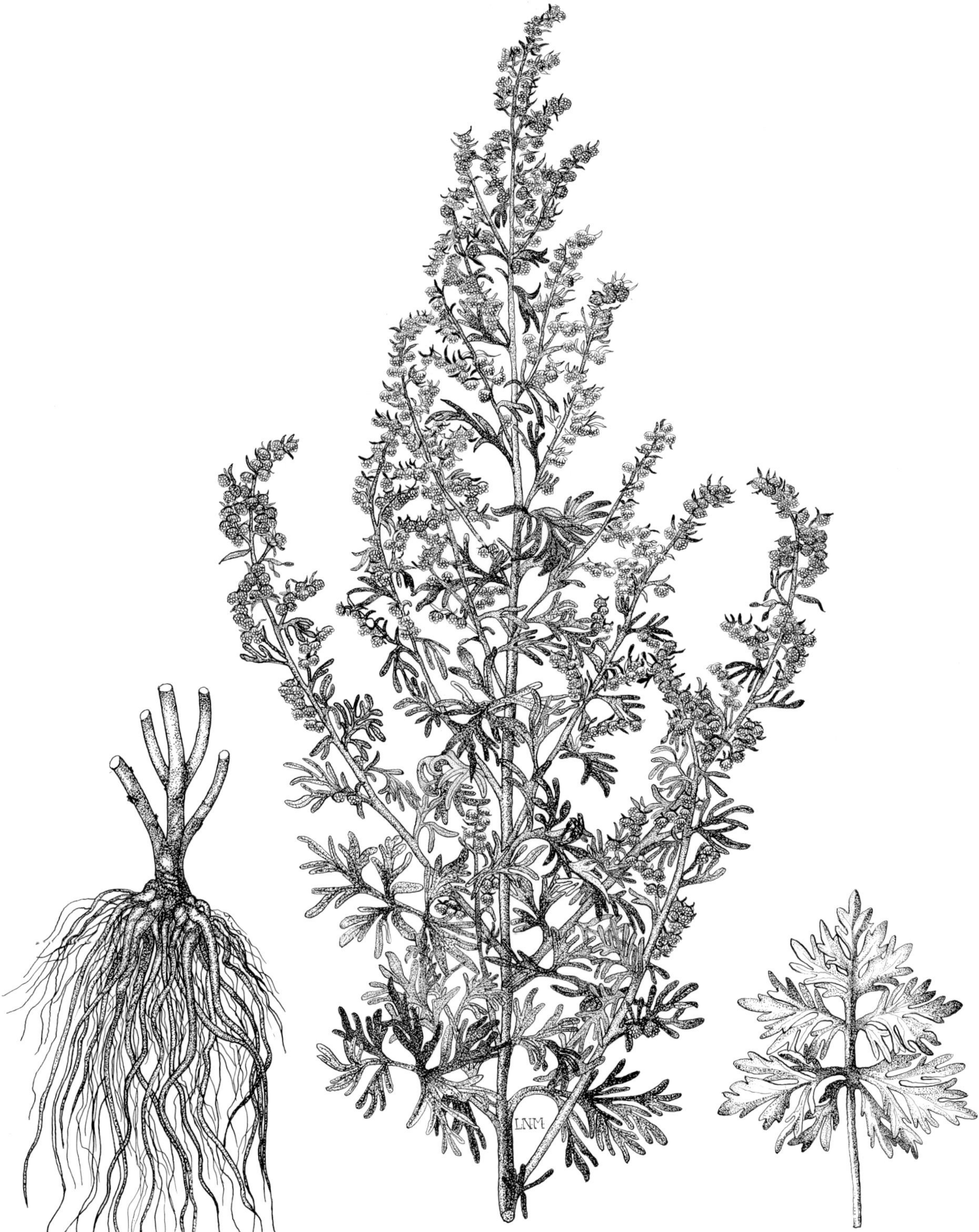
LNM

4 *Calamintha nepeta* (L.) Savi (*Satureja calamintha* (L.) Scheele)

English, calamint savory

Italian, *mentuccia, nepetella*

This mint, a perennial with insignificant small whitish or lilac flowers, growing thirty to eighty centimeters in height, is very common at Pompeii today and in most of the inhabited areas of southern Italy. We know that this mint grew in the Vesuvian area in antiquity because it was found in the carbonized hay at Oplontis.

Today calamint savory is gathered by the Pompeians, boiled in water, and given in this liquid form to *bambini* as a source of vitamins. It is also used in dried bunches in the corners of a room to keep away beetles.

As in modern times, various plants of the mint family were used medicinally in antiquity. It is, however, difficult to identify with accuracy the specific mints mentioned by the ancient authors, who give scant description of the various mints, preferring to concentrate on their medicinal uses. For this reason, identifications in translations of these classical authors are not considered reliable. Pliny uses three different words in discussing mints: (1) *menta,* which may at times refer to *Calamintha nepeta,* (2) *nepeta,* usually identified as *Calamintha nepeta,* and (3) *Mentastrum,* usually horsemint (*Mentha spicata* L. = *M. sylvestris* auct., non L.), which does not apply to our specimen. The only descriptions that Pliny gives of a mint are found in his *Natural History* 19.100, in which he lists *menta* among the plants that "blossom all in a bunch," and in 1.38, where he lists it among the strongest scented garden plants. He gives an extremely long list of medicinal uses for *menta* (*HN* 20.147–151), and a much shorter one for *nepeta* (*HN* 20.158).

Dioscorides gives the medicinal uses for a number of mints including *kalaminthē* (καλαμίνθα), which he says the Romans call *nepeta.* Its leaves were beaten and made into a suppository used as an abortifacient (3.43).

Galen in his treatise *On Simple Drugs according to Temperaments and Faculties* prescribes the oral use of *calamintha* as an abortifacient (*De simplicium medicamentorum temperamentis ac facultatibus* 10. = Kühn ed. 12:6).

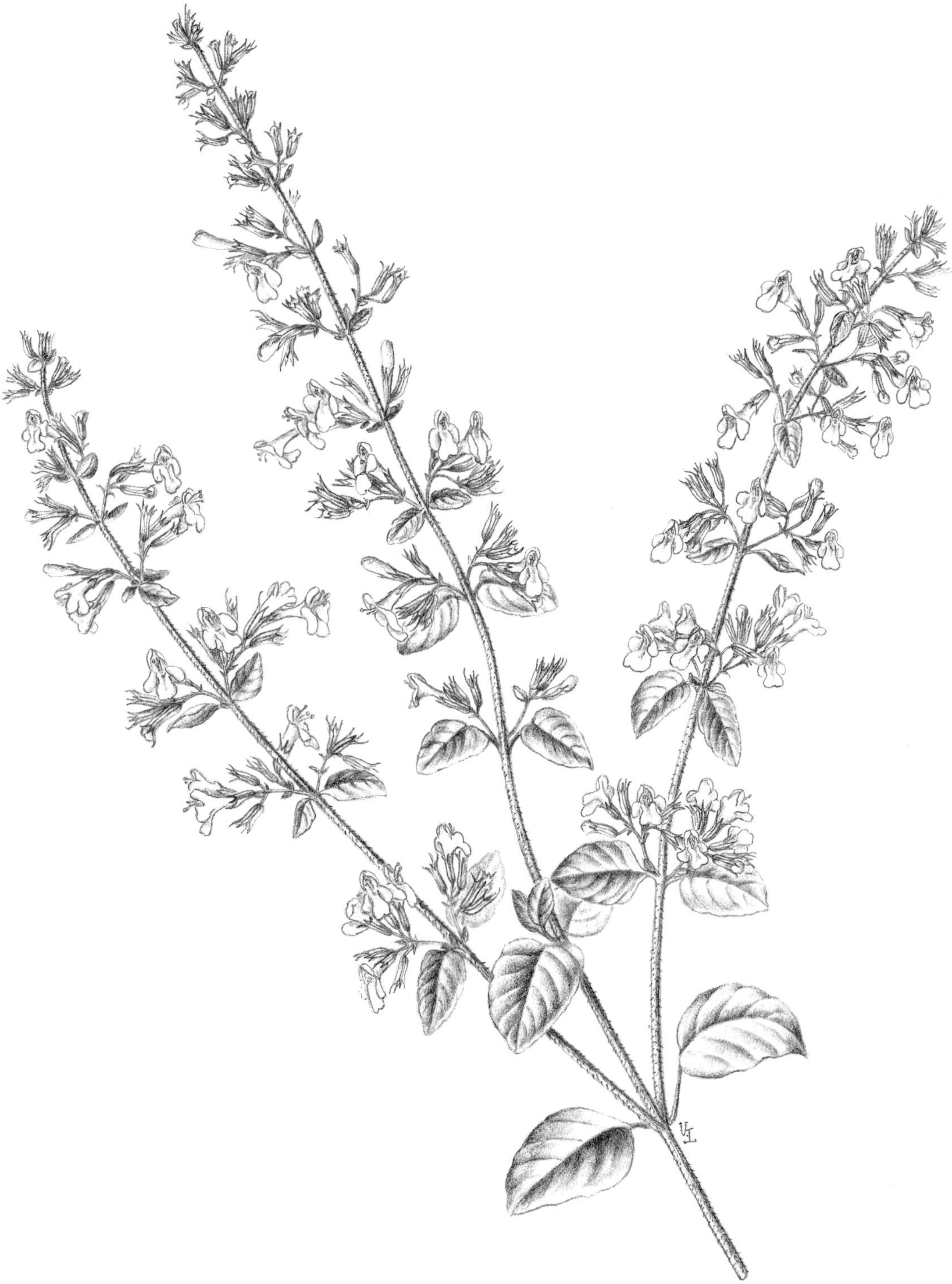

5 *Castanea sativa* Miller

English, European chestnut

Italian, *castagno*

The handsome European chestnut, with its erect trunk and spreading branches, growing to a height of twenty to thirty-five meters, was much valued in antiquity, as it still is today, for its edible nuts and timber. Chestnut pollen was found in various gardens that I excavated. Carbonized chestnuts were found in the excavations, and also in the carbonized hay at Oplontis. The Romans called the chestnut *castanea,* borrowing the Greek name κάσταvος, and this name is incorporated into its modern scientific name.

The chestnut has limited medicinal use in Pompeii today. Chestnuts are boiled together with fennel seeds and laurel leaves, and the liquid is drunk to promote digestion.

Its medicinal use in antiquity was apparently also limited. Pliny, who normally gives a long list of medicinal uses for each plant that he is discussing, says only that chestnuts checked violent diarrhea and encouraged the healthy functioning of the bowels (*HN* 23.150). Dioscorides (1.145) suggests using chestnuts for the same purpose.

Pliny recommended the chestnut for vine props because of the ease "with which it is worked and its obstinate durability" (*HN* 17.147). It did not decay. I found it still used today as props in many Pompeian vineyards, because of its durability.

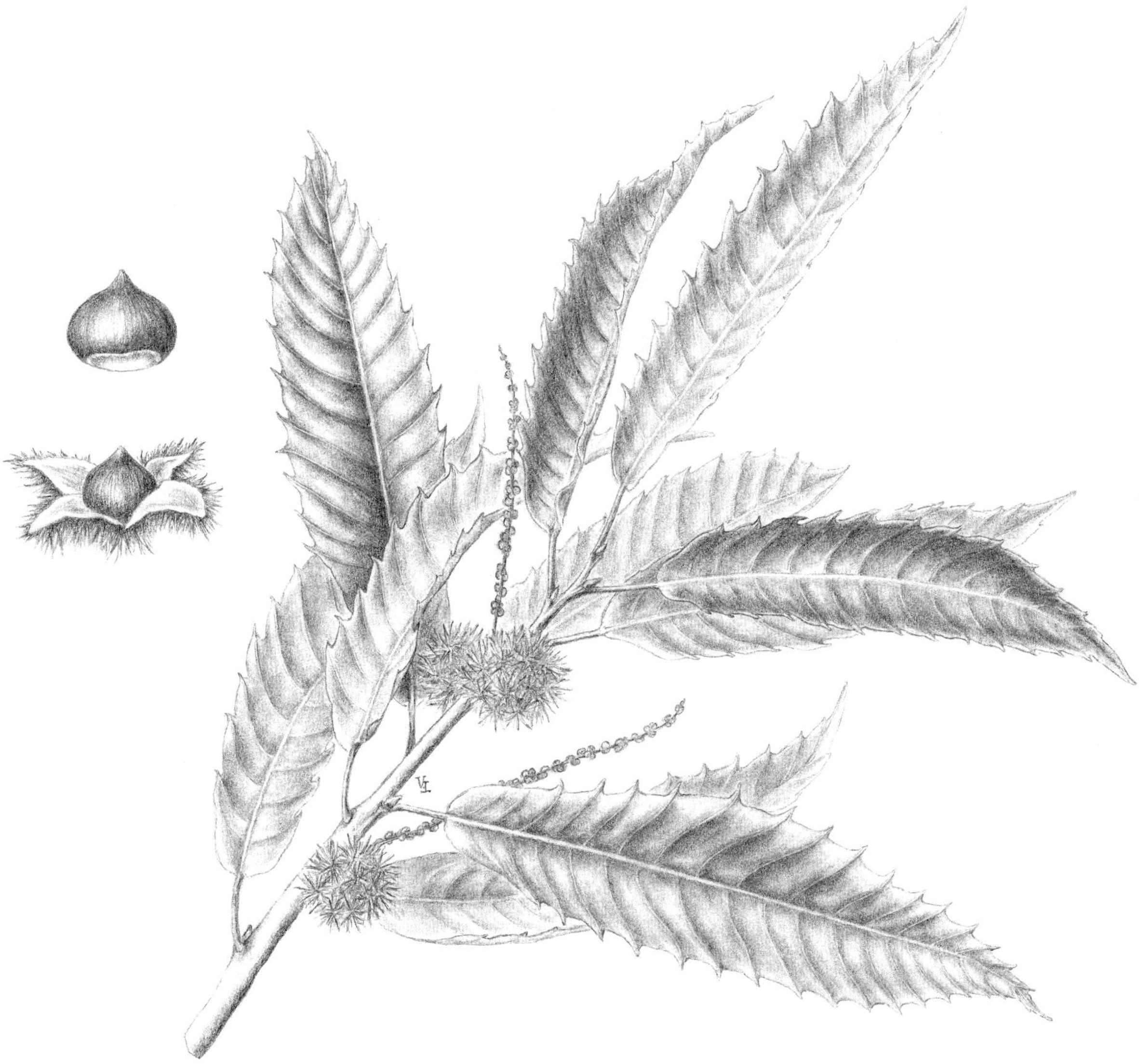

6 *Centranthus ruber* (L.) DC.

English, red valerian

Italian, *valeriana rossa*

Red valerian is an herbaceous perennial, up to eighty centimeters in height, with stems bearing deep rose-colored flowers. It has the characteristic odor found in valerian. It grows in ruins, and on rocks and old walls, flowering from May to August. Valerian grew in the area in antiquity—its pollen was found in the core taken at Lake Avernus. Red valerian is abundant in the excavations today, where large patches of its beautiful flowers are a welcome sight (see Fig. 7).

An infusion of the flowers, or the entire plant, is used at Pompeii to produce sleep, a stronger infusion of the flowers for nervousness or tenseness. The root is used in parts of Italy today for a variety of medicinal purposes. Valerian has lightly narcotic, sedative, and carminative qualities. The sedative Valium gets its name from valerian.

The valerian (*V. phu* L.) known in antiquity by the name *phu* is a close relative and has properties similar to *Centranthus ruber,* which is used medicinally at Pompeii today, and also to *V. officinalis,* which does not grow at Pompeii but is used medicinally elsewhere in Italy.

Pliny (*HN* 21.136) says that the root, pounded or boiled, was given in drink for suffocation of the womb, and for pains in the chest or side. As an emmenagogue, it is taken in wine. Dioscorides (1.10) describes *phu* (φοῦ) as having a stalk a cubit or more in height, with pale white and purple flowers. The upper part of the rhizome is about the thickness of the little finger, with a characteristic odor of a "certain poisonous kind of heaviness." Dioscorides lists much the same medicinal uses as does Pliny.

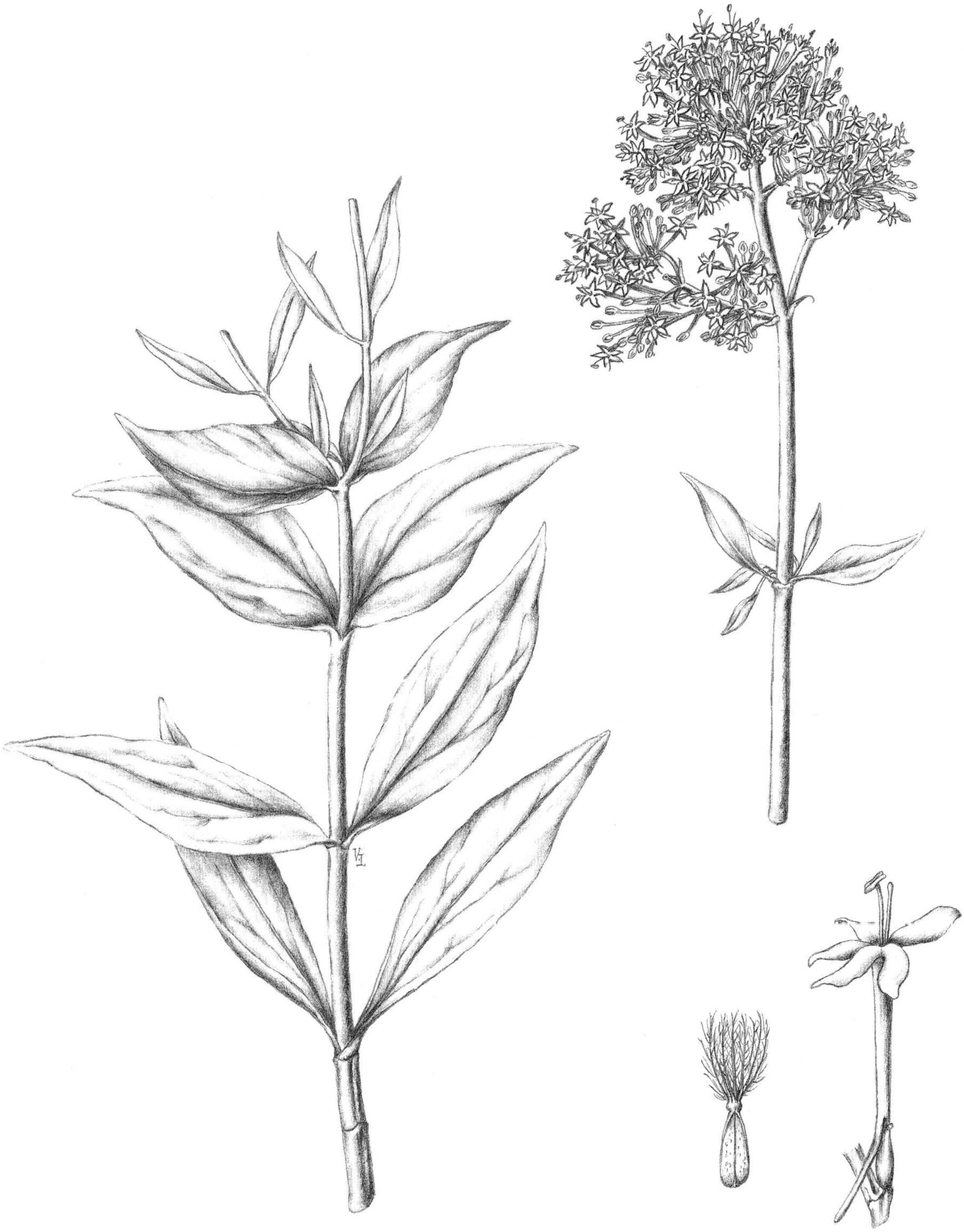

7 *Chamomilla recutita* (L.) Rauschert

English, camomile

Italian, *camomilla*

Enchanted with the shining carpets of little white daisy-like flowers with golden yellow centers (see Fig. 6), as I explored less frequented parts of the excavations, I was curious to learn their name. When told that they were wild camomile, I recalled a name buried deep in the recesses of my mind. This flower must be the source of the famous camomile tea that the adored Peter Rabbit of my childhood was given when he returned home cold and frightened from Mr. McGregor's garden.

I was later to learn that camomile tea made from blossoms gathered at the peak of the summer, dried in the open air in the shade, and boiled in water was extremely popular among the Pompeians as a soothing remedy for nervousness and sleeplessness. But it had other uses. Alone, or when laurel leaves were added, it aided digestion. One of the workmen gave us a bag of dried camomile, which he said had many uses. But he especially recommended boiling the dried plant in water and using it to soothe aching feet. Camomile boiled with laurel leaves is used for digestive problems. This strongly aromatic plant is perhaps the most popular of all medicinal herbs throughout Italy today.

The ancient Romans apparently made less use of this plant. Pliny discusses camomile, but the flower that he refers to cannot be definitely identified. He mentions a plant that they called by many names, including *anthemis* and *chamaemelon* (because its flowers smelled like apples). This confusion can still be found in common names today. Several species of *Anthemis,* which look very much like the camomile, also go by the common name of camomile. Pliny says:

> It (*anthemis,* also called *chamaemelon*) is gathered in spring on thin soils or near foot-paths, and put by for making chaplets. At the same season physicians also make into lozenges the pounded leaves, as well as the blossom and the root. All three are mixed and given in doses of one drachma for bites of every kind of snake. Taken in drink they bring away the dead fetus, are emmenagogues and diuretic. (*HN* 22.53–54)

Dioscorides (3.154), who also calls it *anthemis* (ἀνθεμίς), but says some call it *chamaimēlon* (χαμαίμηλον), gives much the same medicinal uses as Pliny.

Galen, as at Pompeii today, prescribed it for sleeplessness (*De simpl. med. temp. ac fac.* 6.1.45 = Kühn ed. 11:832).

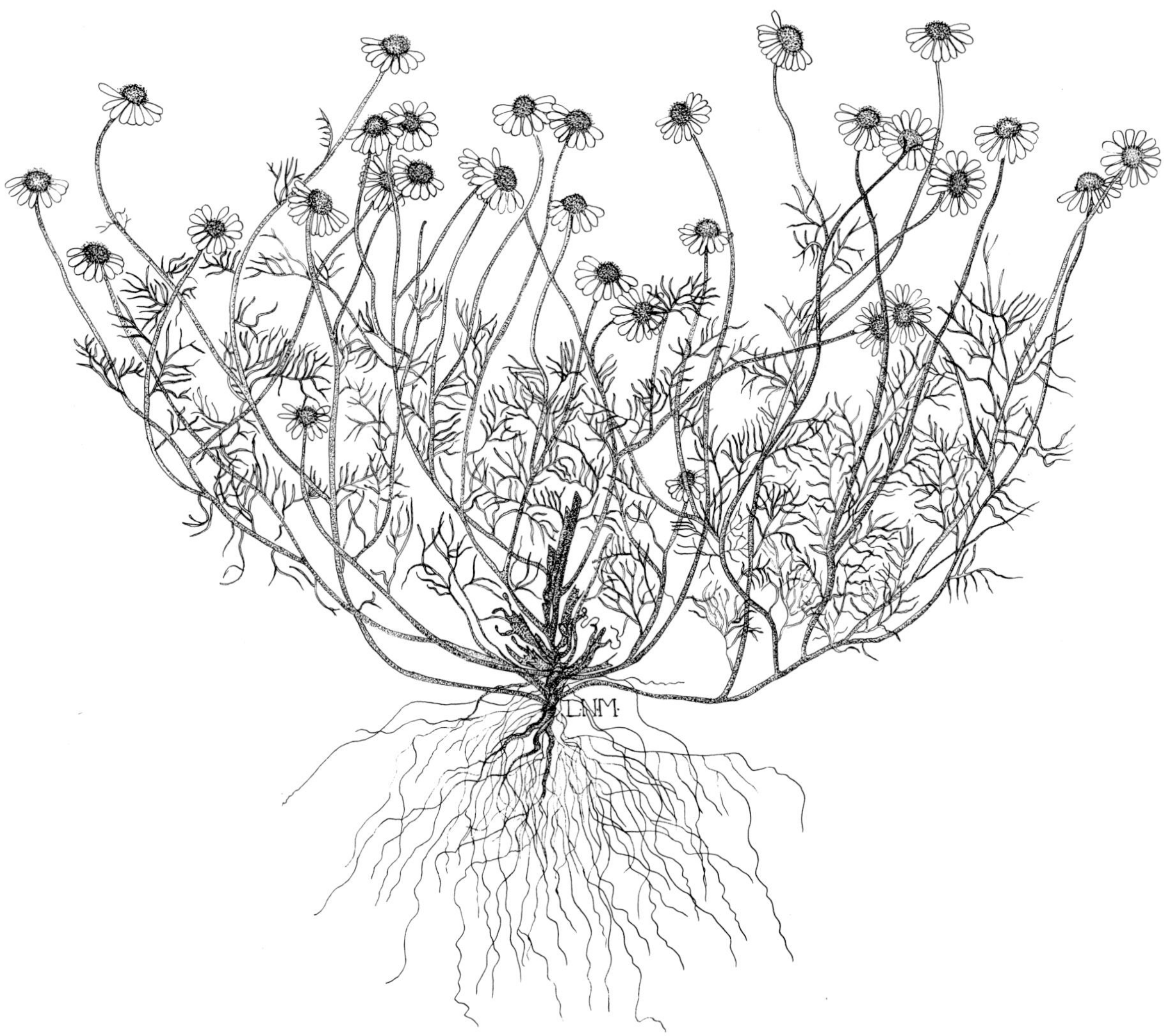
LNM

8 *Cichorium intybus* L.

ENGLISH, CHICORY

Italian, *cicoria, radicchio*

Chicory is a tall perennial, 30 to 120 centimeters in height, with tough green stems and spreading branches, and bright blue flowers in a few flowered heads. It grows in uncultivated land around the Mediterranean and is very common in the excavated areas at Pompeii.

I found chicory used medicinally for only one purpose at Pompeii. Boiled in water, it is highly regarded as a specific for stomach ailments.

In antiquity an infusion of chicory was likewise used for stomach problems, as well as for many other ailments. Pliny recommended chicory (*cichorium*) for stomach problems; it was also a laxative, as well as a specific for jaundice and for liver, kidney, and bladder problems; it helped the purgation of women and even expelled the dead fetus. The list is long. Pliny adds, "So great indeed are its health-giving properties that some call it *chreston* (useful), others *pancration* (almighty)" (*HN* 20.74).

Dioscorides (2.160) refers to chicory (κιχόριον) as a wild plant which is narrow-leaved and bitter. He, too, recommends it as very good for the stomach.

The dried roots of chicory are used today commercially, roasted and mixed with coffee to adulterate it; this gives it the characteristic bitter flavor liked by some. But when a Neapolitan tastes bad coffee, he says, "What is this, chicory?" During World War II chicory was used as a coffee substitute. Chicory is one of the bitter herbs used to make a soup which is traditionally eaten with the paschal lamb.

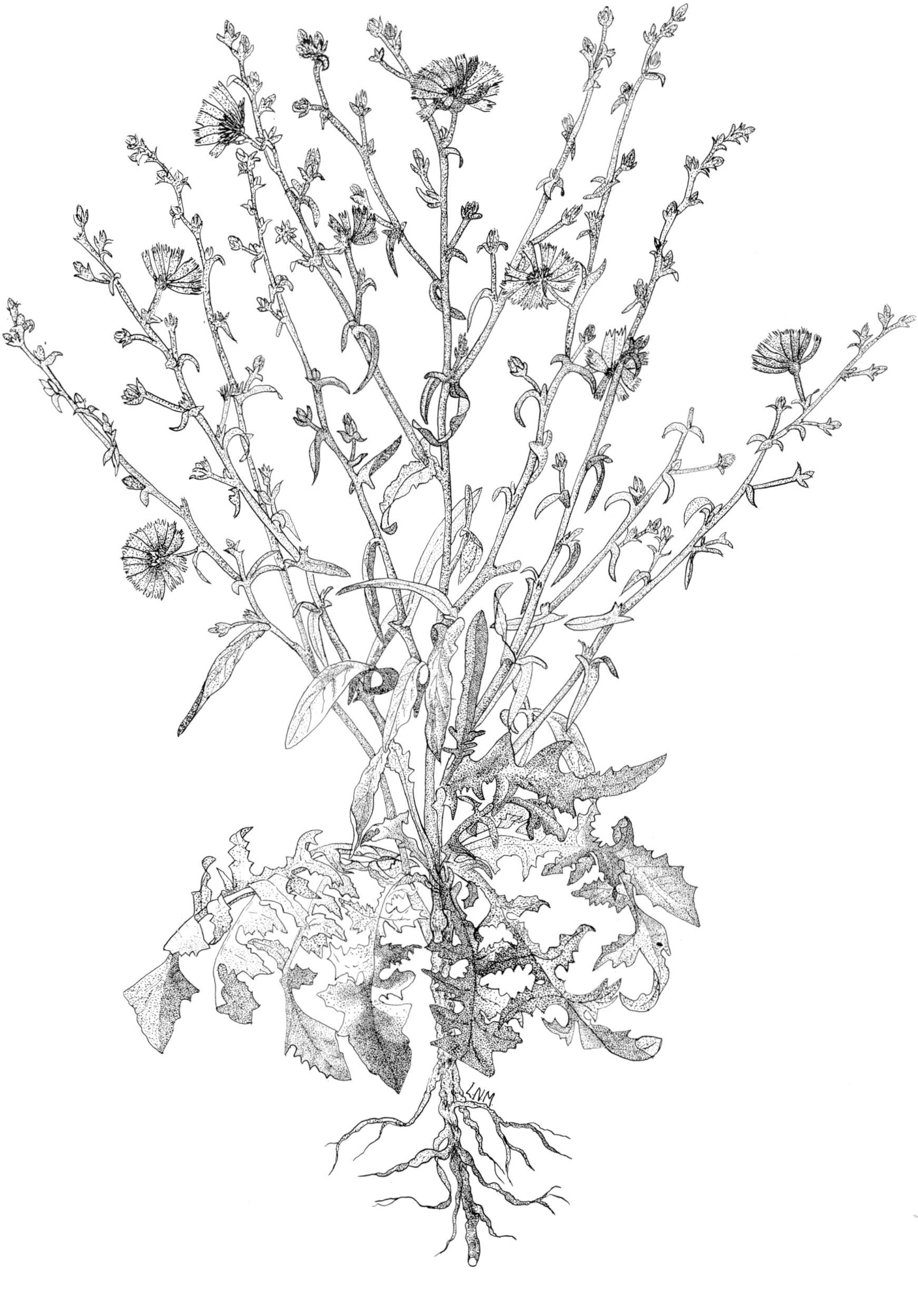
LNM

9 *Citrus limon* (L.) Burm. f.

ENGLISH, LEMON

Italian, *limone*

Lemon juice is used in the Pompeii area as a remedy for stomach and intestinal ailments, especially diarrhea. It is also used as a mouthwash, and as a gargle for sore throat. The country people apply lemon leaves on wounds, boils, and abscesses to cure them. Women wash their hands with lemon juice mixed with flour to make them smooth and white.

A tonic (and a not unpleasant drink) recommended for stomach ailments has as its basic ingredient the thinnest lemon peel, without any white, to which is added three hundred grams of sugar, five hundred to six hundred grams of water, and various flavorings.

It is difficult to identify any passages from the ancient authors that might refer to the lemon due to the absence in antiquity of a terminology to designate the different species of citrus fruit. Tolkowsky (p. xii) points out:

> Due to the fact that the citron was the first citrus fruit known to the classical world, the name given to it by the Latin writers, *citrus,* was subsequently extended to all other plants, which, as they successively found their way into the Mediterranean world, were, because of their similarity in botanical character, felt to be closely related to the citron itself.

Linnaeus later also used *Citrus* as the scientific name for the entire genus.

Because the lemon lacked a Latin name, it has been believed that it was unknown in antiquity and must have arrived late in Europe. But the Romans clearly knew the lemon and painted lemon trees with accurately portrayed fruit, as, for example, in the two rooms in the House of the Fruit Orchard (I.ix.5) at Pompeii which picture fruit trees. The Romans also distinguished the lemon and citron as two very different fruits, as a mosaic of ca. A.D. 100 in the Terme Museum at Rome (inv. no. 58596) clearly shows. The carbonized root of a lemon tree identified in my excavations in the sculpture garden of the villa of Poppaea at Oplontis shows that the lemon was grown in the area. Dioscorides recommends the Persian or the Median apple (names by which the citron was first known to the Romans) for stomach problems (1.164) and the juice as a mouthwash (1.166), uses similar to that of the lemon today.

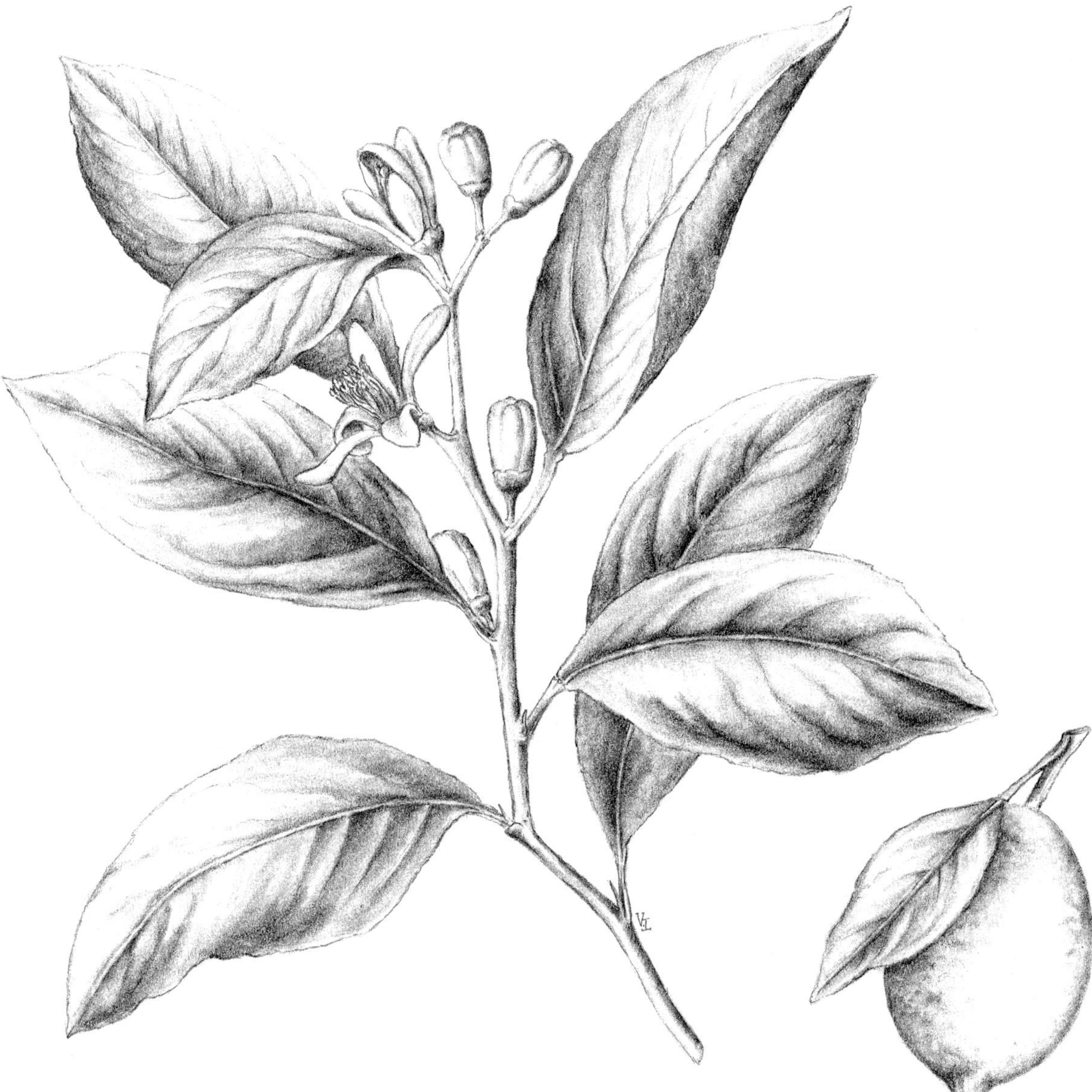

10 *Cyclamen hederifolium* Aiton (*C. neapolitanum* Ten.)

English, cyclamen

Italian, *ciclamino*

One of the aged workmen at Pompeii was a fertile source of information about medicinal plants. One year, just before returning to the United States, I asked him if he had told me about every plant that he used. "Everything that grows at Pompeii," he answered. "But there is the potato at Stabiae." It seems that it had saved his life. I assured him that Stabiae was of equal interest to me. It too had been covered by the eruption of Vesuvius. He then recounted the dramatic story of how he had been in the hospital, dying of a terrible infection of the head. Medicine was of no avail. But he told the doctors that the potato from Stabiae would cure him. They agreed to get it, and prepared it according to his instructions, grating it and packing it into his nostrils. Then suddenly all the poison gushed out, and he was healed. I asked him the name of this miraculous cure. He knew it only as *la patata* (the potato). I asked him if it had a flower, and he said it was of no consequence, somewhat like a violet. I asked if he could get me some potatoes. We sent some "potatoes" to Dr. Meyer, who had them planted in the greenhouse at the U.S. National Arboretum. When the "potato" bloomed, it was the lovely Neapolitan cyclamen. Some years later, when I excavated the gardens at Hadrian's villa at Tivoli, near Rome, it was a great joy to find jewel-like patches of these cyclamen in bloom.

It was exciting to discover that the ancient Romans had used this plant in the same way that it had been used to dramatically cure the Pompeian workman. Pliny (*HN* 25.134) says that the root of the cyclamen (*cyclaminos*) pushed into the nostrils clears the head. He gives an interesting description of the cyclamen:

> The plant has smaller, darker, and thinner leaves than those of ivy, with no corners but with white spots; the stem is short and hollow, the blossom purple, the root so broad that it might be taken for that of the turnip, and having a dark skin. It grows in shaded spots, is called by our countrymen *tuber terrae* [earth truffle], and ought to be grown in every home if it is true that wherever it grows no evil spells do any harm. They call it "amulet," and say that if it is added to wine intoxication comes at once. (*HN* 25.114–115)

Pliny gives many other medicinal uses for the root of the cyclamen. Theophrastus (9.9.1) says the root and the juice of the cyclamen (κυκλάμινος) are used as medicine. Dioscorides (2.194) says that the juice [of the root] put into the nostrils with honey purges the head. Both Scribonius (7) and Galen, in his *Commentary I on the Hippocratic Book on Body Fluids* (*in Hippoc.* 12 = Kühn ed. 16:147), also recommended cleaning the nostrils with cyclamen juice to clear the head. Pliny (*HN* 21.51) adds that the cyclamen flower was used in making chaplets.

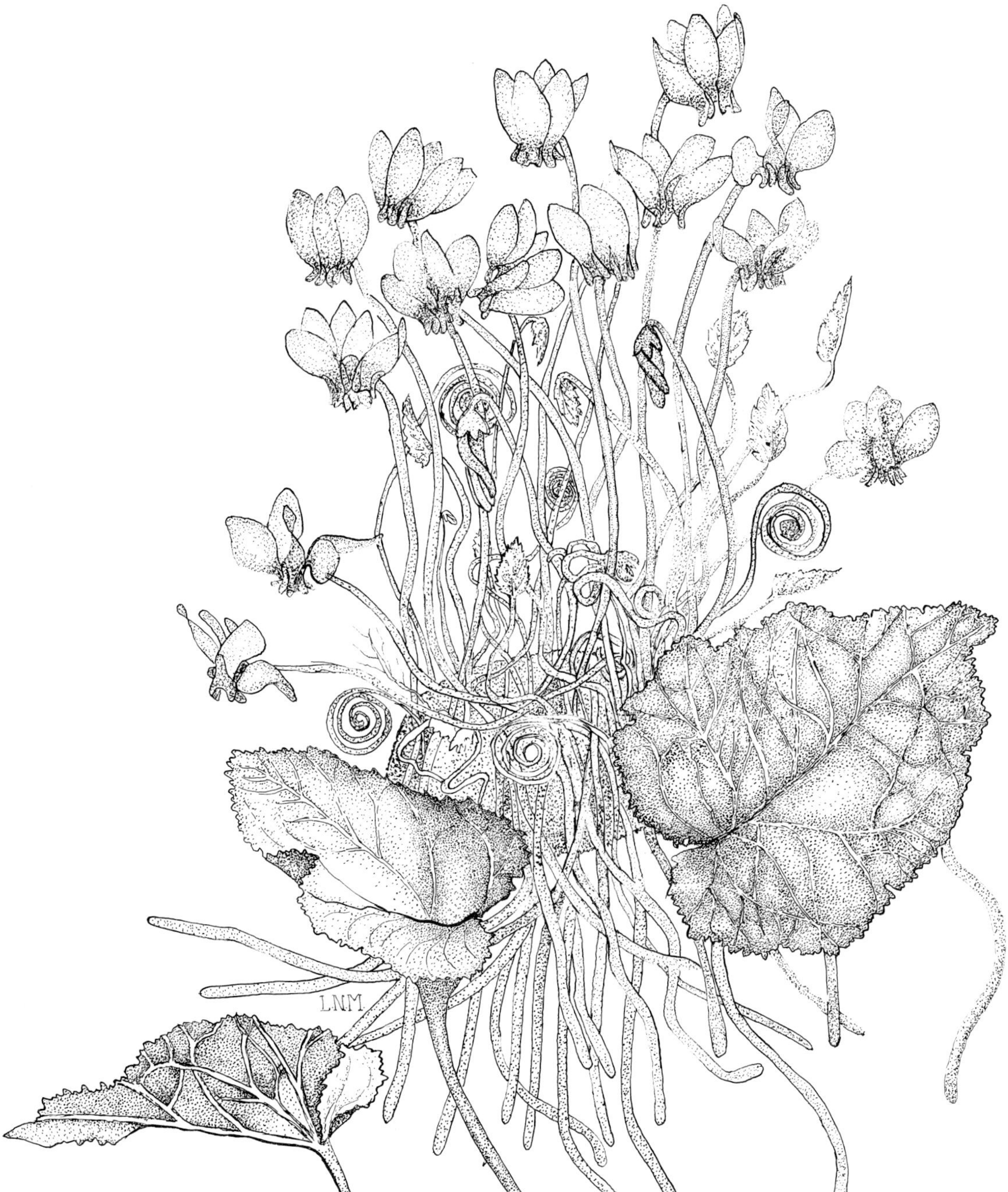
LNM

11 *Cynodon dactylon* (L.) Pers.

English, Bermuda grass

Italian, *gramigna, erba canina, capriola*

Bermuda grass is a low greyish-green creeping, invasive perennial grass that grows rapidly. The inflorescence consists of a thin culm with several (3–6) narrow finger-like spikes, which gives it its name. Its stout creeping stems root at the joints, bearing short leafy shoots that grow together in a mat. When a cultivated field is invaded, it is very difficult to eradicate. But this same quality explains its wide use today as a lawn grass. Not surprisingly this invasive grass was found in the carbonized hay at Oplontis.

The rhizome has a variety of medicinal uses at Pompeii. It is used as a diuretic and to stimulate the circulation of the blood. It is also used in combination with other plants. Boiled in water with polygonum, tender blackberry tips, and fennel and sweetened with sugar, the liquid is used hot for colds, and cold to aid digestion. When the rhizomes of Bermuda grass are boiled together with the roots of the common mallow and knot-grass, the resulting liquid can be used to alleviate stomach problems.

Pliny gives a good description of Bermuda grass (*gramen*), which he calls the very commonest of plants (*HN* 24.178, 19.98). This humble grass had been held in high esteem since early times; the greatest honor among the Romans was a crown made of Bermuda grass, for it could be "voted only by the whole army and only to him who had rescued it" (*HN* 22.7). In former days the crown was

> made from green grass pulled up from the site where the besieged men had been relieved by some one. For in old times it was the most solemn token of defeat for the conquered to present grass to their conquerors, for to do so meant that they withdrew from their land, from the very soil that nurtured them and even from means of burial. (*HN* 22.8)

Pliny lists those who had received this coveted crown from earliest times down to his own day (*HN* 22.9–13). He gives numerous medicinal uses of Bermuda grass: it prevents vomiting, checks looseness of the bowels, prevents bleeding, cures snake bites, and has many other uses. It was used alone and in combinations (*HN* 24.179–181). He refers to this grass only once as *dactylon* (finger), a name incorporated into its modern scientific name, when he speaks of pointed grasses: "when on each head there are at most five points they call it finger-grass (*dactylon*)" (*HN* 24.182).

Dioscorides (4.30) also gives a good description of this grass, which he calls *agrostis* (ἄγρωστις) and cites its medicinal use for a variety of ailments, including ulcers of the bladder and gallstones.

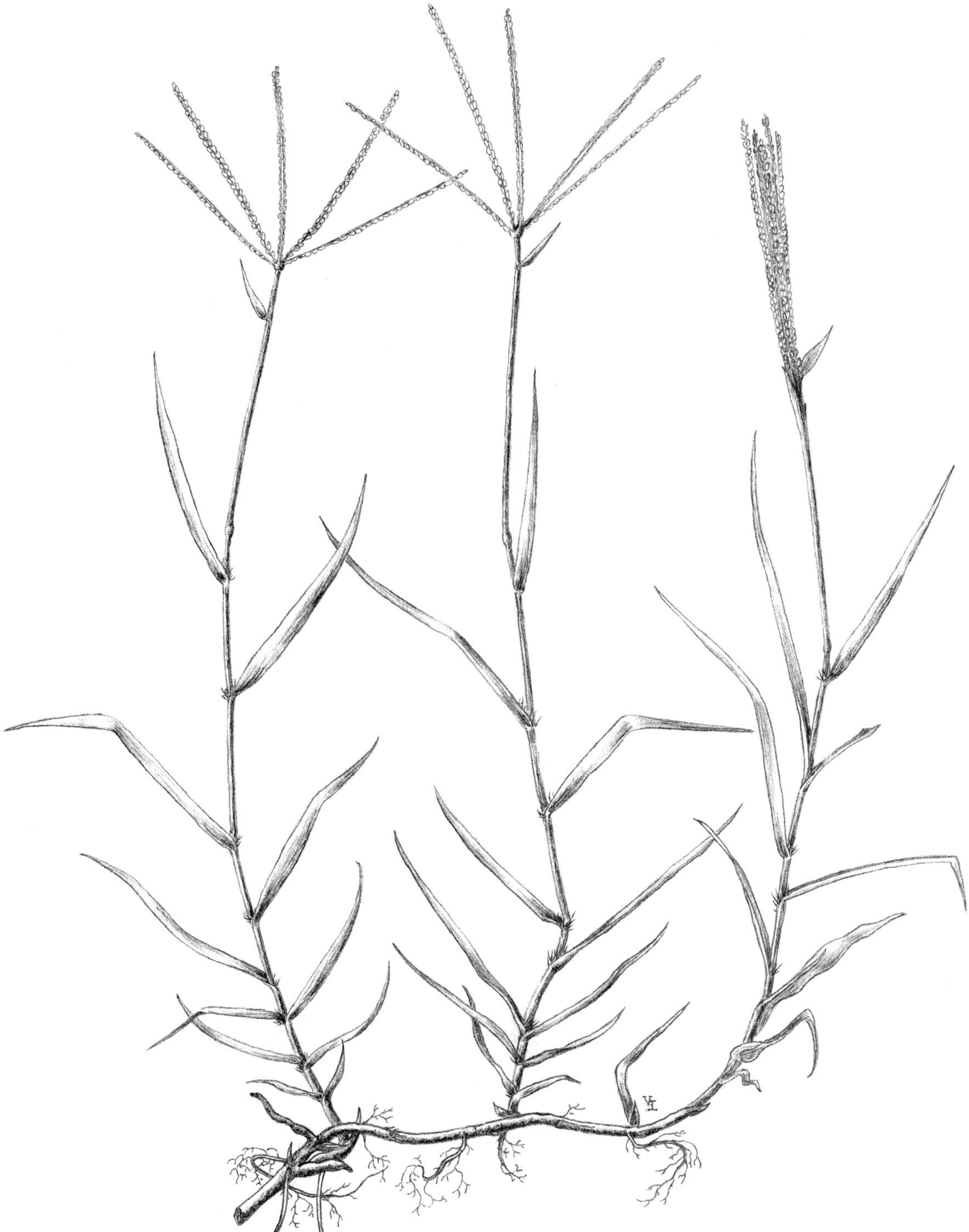

12 *Delphinium halteratum* Sibth. & Sm.

English, larkspur

Italian, *speronella, sprone di cavaliere*

This larkspur, a low-growing annual with spikes of blue-violet flowers and spurs longer than the colored sepals, grows fifteen to thirty-five centimeters in height and is found in fields and arid places around the Mediterranean. It can be seen throughout the ruins at Pompeii.

The Pompeians boil this larkspur in water, which is used to stop any hemorrhaging that occurs after childbirth. At one time the seeds were used as an emetic and a drastic purgative. The plant is very poisonous, and today at Pompeii oil extracted from the seeds is used chiefly as an insecticide.

Pliny mentions only one larkspur (*staphis* or *astaphis agria*), known botanically as *Delphinium staphisagria* L. (*HN* 23.17–18). All species of *Delphinium* have similar properties and are poisonous. He, too, prescribes its use as an insecticide: the stones (seeds) pounded rid the head of lice, as well as the rest of the body, and also cure itch scab. A decoction in vinegar assuages toothache and ear ailments. He advises against using the seeds as a purge, as was done in years past in modern Pompeii, or to dry phlegm in the mouth. Pounded flowers taken in wine counteract the poisons of serpents, but he warns against using the seed.

Dioscorides (4.156) gives a similar description of this larkspur (σταφίς ἄγρια) and more medicinal uses. He does not share Pliny's concern about using it as a purge, or to dry phlegm in the mouth. He also recommends it for toothache. He describes another larkspur, which he calls *delphinion* (δελφίνιον) (3.84), as bearing seeds in pods that resemble millet; the seeds taken in wine are recommended for one use only, scorpion bites.

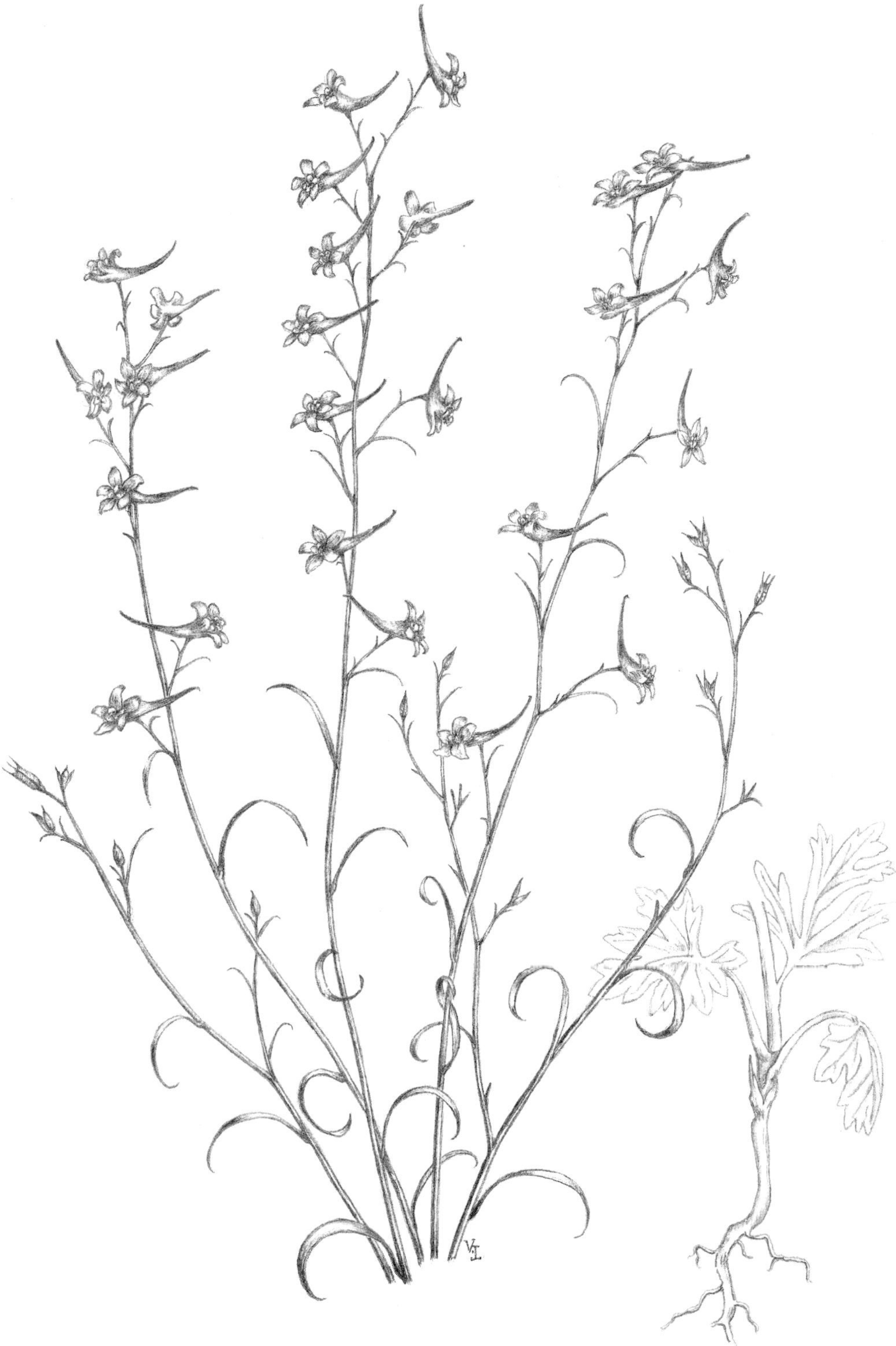

13 *Diplotaxis tenuifolia* (L.) DC.

ENGLISH, WALL ROCKET

Italian, *rucola, ruchetta selvatica*

Rocket is an herbaceous annual of the mustard family, branched from the base, thirty to sixty centimeters high, leaves with long and narrow segments, and bright yellow, long-pedicelled flowers. It grows in waste ground and stony places and along roadsides.

I first saw rocket growing as a weed in the House of Pansa (VI.vi.1/12), where it was pointed out to me by the gardener, who told me that the leaves were eaten in salads at Pompeii. It is consumed in the spring to purify the blood. Guarrera (p. 61) notes that it is a source of vitamin C.

Rocket was also known in antiquity as a salad plant. Pliny (*HN* 19.117,154) lists a rocket, which he calls *eruca,* among the kitchen garden plants that grow equally well in summer and winter, as does Columella (11.3.14). The Roman name *eruca* was incorporated into the scientific name of another rocket, *Eruca sativa* L., a close relative of *Diplotaxis tenuifolia. Eruca sativa* grows wild but is also cultivated as a salad plant, for its somewhat larger leaves. Both plants are known today as rocket (*ruchetta* in Italy), and it is quite possible that the Romans also referred to both plants by a single name.

Pliny recommends mixing rocket, which has aphrodisiac qualities, with lettuce as a salad, so that the excessive chilliness of the lettuce may be mitigated by an equal amount of heat (*HN* 19.155). He also gives a long list of the medicinal uses of rocket seed: it cures poison from scorpions and the shrew-mouse; it keeps off body parasites; mixed with honey, it removes spots from the face, and freckles when this mixture is applied with vinegar; taken in wine, it hardens the feelings of those about to be flogged. It was regarded as such a pleasant seasoning for food that the Greeks called it "good broth" (*euzōmon,* εὔζωμον). Slightly pounded rocket restores clearness of vision to the eye; it is a good cough medicine for babies (*HN* 20.125–126).

Dioscorides (2.170) also refers to a rocket (εὔζωμον) which has been identified with *Eruca sativa* as an aphrodisiac, and says it is good for digestion. See also the Roman satirist Martial (*Epigrams* 3.75). The Roman poet Horace (*Satires* 2.8.51) speaks of a sauce improved by the addition of green rocket.

In *The Roman Cookery Book* (*De re coquinaria*) attributed to Apicius, rocket is used in a sauce for boiled crane or duck (6.2.6), in a dressing for grey mullet (9.10.7), and the seeds in a sauce for boiled boar (8.1.8). Rocket seed is included in a medicine that aids digestion, prevents colds, and is a laxative (1.13).

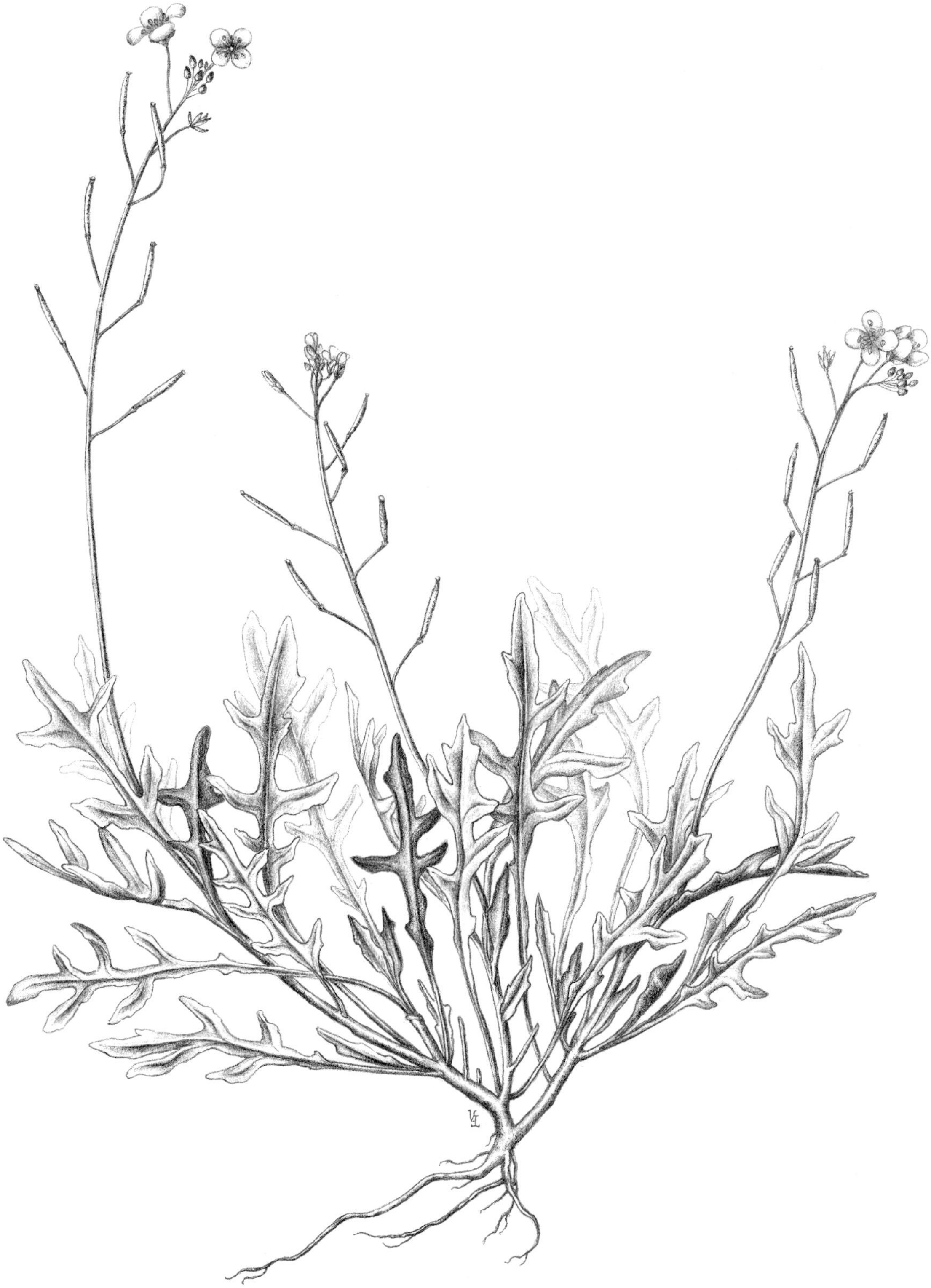

14 *Eucalyptus camaldulensis* Dehnh.

English, eucalyptus, gum tree

Italian, *eucalipto*

The eucalyptus tree is a newcomer to Pompeii, having been brought to the west from Australia in the nineteenth century. But the modern Pompeians have discovered its virtues as a medicinal plant. It is known at Pompeii by its Neapolitan name, *calipso.* At Pompeii five leaves boiled in one liter of water are a specific for constipation. If the ailment is more serious, boil the five leaves in a half liter of water. For a cold, boil seventy or eighty leaves in water until the foliage is soft, and strain through a cloth. Heat the liquid and inhale the vapor to cure the cold. For fever, bruise a bunch of leaves in one-fourth of a liter of alcohol. Let stand for twenty-four hours. Use as a massage in the morning and evening. I was told that this was *una medicina grandiosa.* A priest at Pompeii told me that he took it regularly for his diabetes.

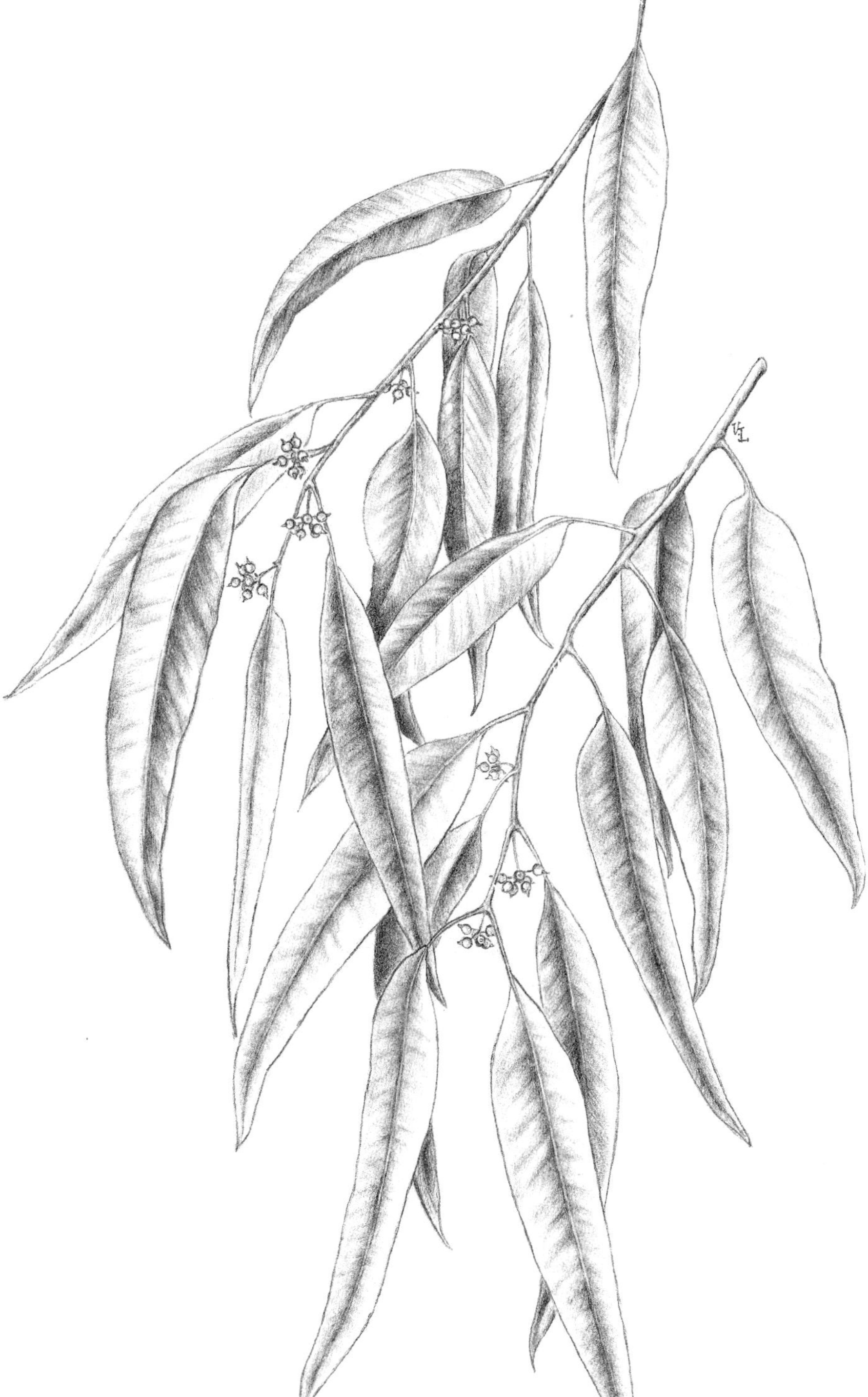

15 *Ficus carica* L.

ENGLISH, FIG

Italian, *fico*

Figs were among the most highly esteemed fruits in ancient Campania, as they still are today. Among the many joys of working in Italy were the fresh figs in season, generously given to us by our workmen from their own trees, and also eagerly sought from the fruit vendors. Carbonized figs were found in the ancient shops, and remains of burned figs were identified in the refuse of sacrifices at the temple of Isis.

But I learned that the fig is also valued for its medicinal properties. The milky juice obtained from the leaves, broken branches, or green fruit, if applied several times a day to warts, softens them, and they can then be removed if bathed in hot water. The milky juice applied to sunburn relieves it in a short time. The fruit is important as a laxative. It is also added to barley water to make a refreshing tonic.

Pliny (*ficus, HN* 23.117–130) and Dioscorides (συκῆ, 1.183) report many medicinal uses of the fig. They give an almost endless list of cures effected by using the milky juice, or the fruit prepared in different ways. Pliny, like the modern Pompeian, recommends the fig to remove warts, and both authors list it as a laxative, as does Celsus (2.29.1). Among the various external uses of the fig, Celsus (5.28.14.E) recommends a fig boiled in water to remove a certain kind of wart. Scribonius (66) uses dried figs in a decoction to treat abscesses in the throat.

Soranus (1.61–62), who says it is much better not to conceive than to destroy the embryo, lists a suppository made of dried figs among his contraceptives. There is clear evidence in the ancient sources that the Greeks and Romans had knowledge of herbal means of both birth control and abortion and that they were aware of the difference between the two. Soranus states this difference clearly (1.60):

> A contraceptive differs from an abortion, for the first does not let conception take place, while the latter destroys what has been conceived. Let us, therefore, call the one "abortive" and the other "contraceptive."

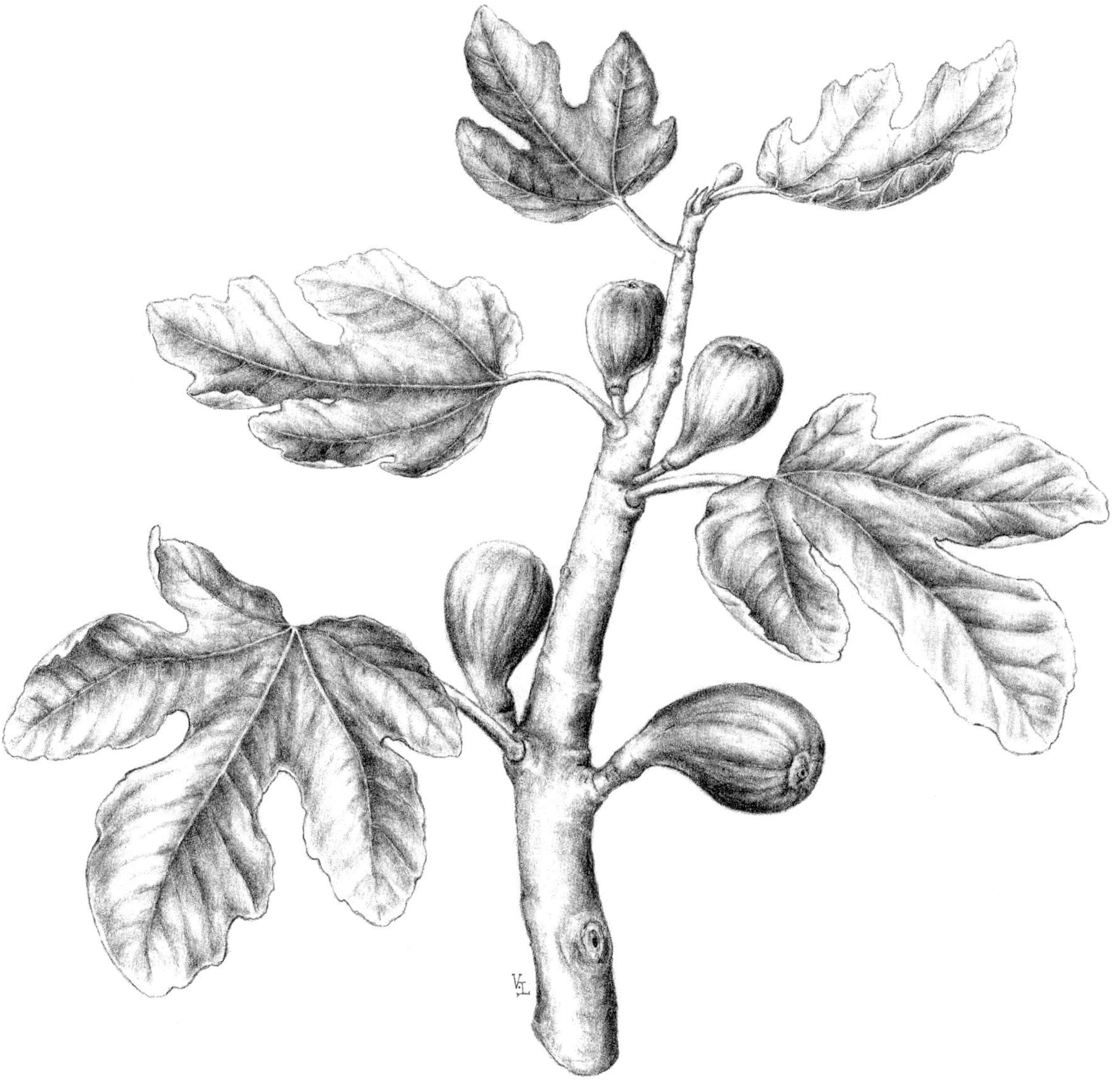
VL

16 *Foeniculum vulgare* Miller

English, fennel

Italian, *finocchio, finocchietto*

Fennel, an aromatic perennial, three to four meters in height, with fine, feathery leaves and umbels of small, intense yellow flowers, grows luxuriously in excavated areas at Pompeii. Women living in the excavations recommended it, boiled in water, for digestive problems. Dry fennel seeds taken in the mouth after eating were recommended for stomach ailments. When the plant is boiled in water along with Bermuda grass, knotgrass, and tender blackberry tips, and sweetened, the resulting liquid can be drunk cold for digestive problems, or hot for colds. A mixture of fennel seeds boiled with laurel leaves and chestnuts is used for digestive problems.

Pliny gives many medicinal uses of fennel (*feniculum*), but he is most interested in it as an eye medicine.

> Fennel has been made famous . . . by serpents, which taste it to cast off their old skin and with its juice improve their eyesight. Consequently it has been inferred that by fennel juice especially can dimness of human vision also be removed. This juice is collected when the stem is swelling to bud, dried in the sun and applied in honey as an ointment. The most esteemed is gathered in Spain from the tear-drops of the plant. (*HN* 20.254)

Fennel had various medicinal uses in combination with other herbs. Pliny reports "a very famous preparation" used to counteract the poison of venomous animals. The preparation must have been considered of great importance for, as we have seen, the formula with exact measurements was carved in verse on a stone in the temple of Asclepius in Cos. It contains among other things fennel seeds, aniseed, trefoil seed, wild thyme, juice of all-heal, and parsley—all ground together, sieved, and then kneaded with the best wine obtainable into lozenges, to be taken with wine (*HN* 20.264).

Celsus recommends fennel to relieve flatulence (2.26.2) and as a diuretic (2.31), and the seeds used externally as a repressant and refrigerant to allay fever (2.33.2). Dioscorides (3.81) gives even more medicinal uses of fennel (μάραθρον): as a specific for stomach problems (as in Pompeii today), for bladder problems, fever, snake and dog bites, and eye problems. The famous Battle of Marathon, in which the Greeks defeated the Persians in 490 B.C., takes its name from the plain on the coast of Attica, so named because it was overgrown by fennel (μάραθον, Attic Greek form).

Scribonius prescribes a liquid medication that includes the juice of fennel for eye problems (cataracts) (38); fennel seeds in medications to treat gout in the feet (159, 160); and fennel seeds in two elaborate medications to treat snake or rabid dog bite (176, 177).

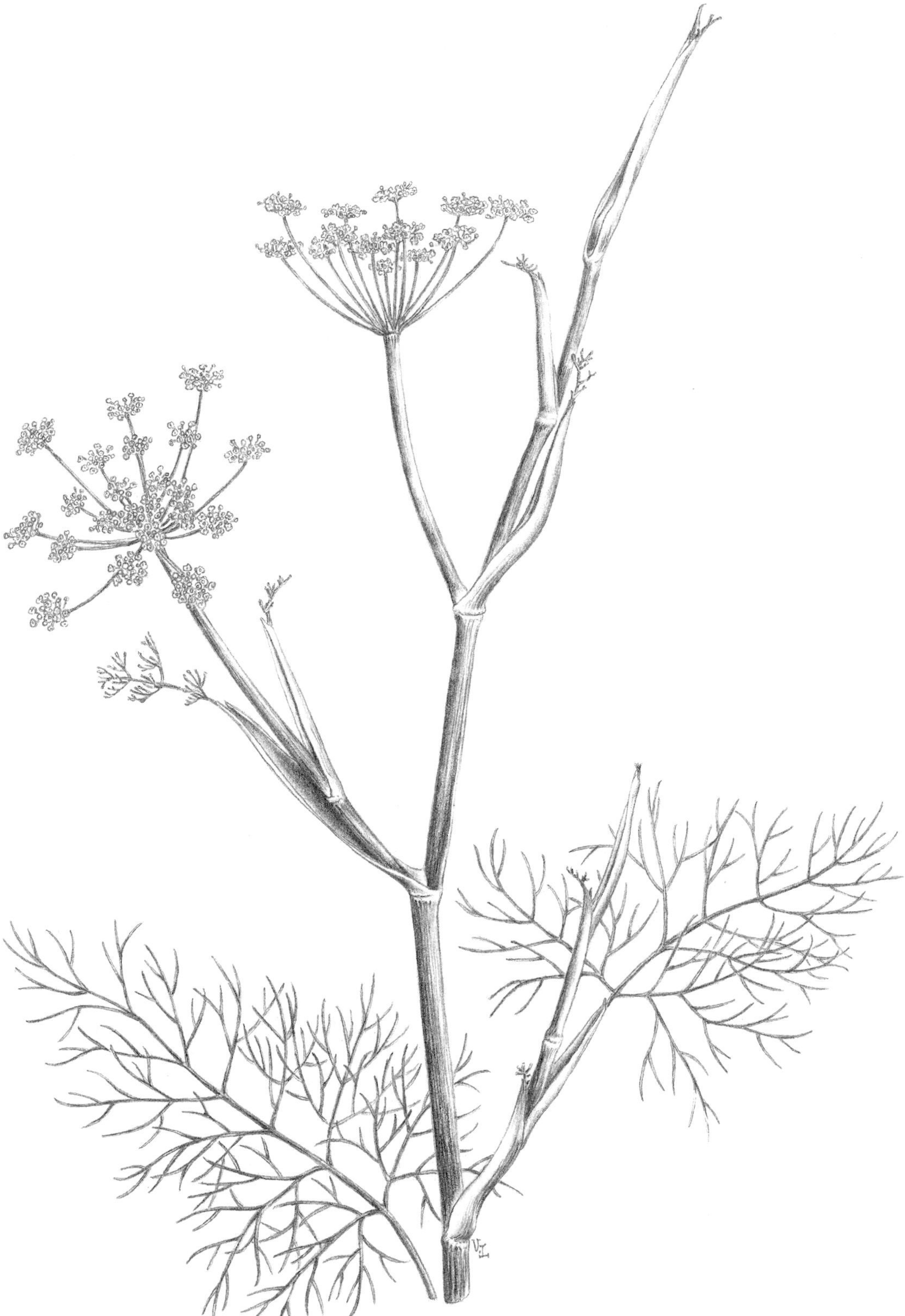

17 *Hordeum vulgare* L.

English, six-rowed barley

Italian, *orzo*

Barley water, made by putting a handful of barley in one liter of water and then skimming off the scum, is considered a refreshing tonic at Pompeii. The Pompeians tell me it is better if dry figs and sugar are added. This tonic is also recommended for children.

Six-rowed barley was a popular crop in the area in antiquity, as is shown by the carbonized barley from the excavations now on display in the Naples Museum, at Pompeii, and at Herculaneum. A graffito scratched on a *villa rustica* in the *fondo Juliana* at Boscoreale records the barley raised there.

Pliny (*HN* 22.134–136) gives a number of medicinal uses of barley (*hordeum*). He says that Hippocrates devoted a whole volume to praising the virtues of ptisan (barley water) (see the Hippocratic Corpus, *Regimen in Acute Diseases,* especially chap. 10). Dioscorides (2.108) also recommends this nourishing drink. He gives various medicinal uses of barley (κριθή). Celsus recommends a decoction of pearl barley (*ptisana*) for a soothing enema (2.12.1.D; 3.19.5); for diarrhea, vomiting, or thirst connected with cholera, wine sprinkled with barley porridge (*polenta*) or mint applied to the nostrils; later a drink of diluted wine with barley porridge added to give the patient strength (4.18.3–4); barley bread as a laxative (2.29.1); and barley meal (*hordeacia farina*) for making poultices (3.27.2.C).

Soranus uses barley in various prescriptions, including barley juice in a mixture to clean the newborn (2.13); barley juice and honey water dropped in a baby's mouth, for tonsillitis (2.50); in a poultice for severe skin ulcerations in children (2.52); liquid barley gruel as food in difficult labor (4.7). Galen, too, speaks of the virtues of ptisan in his treatise *On Ptisan* (*De ptisana* 1–6 = Kühn ed. 6:816–831 = *CMG* 5.4.2:455–463).

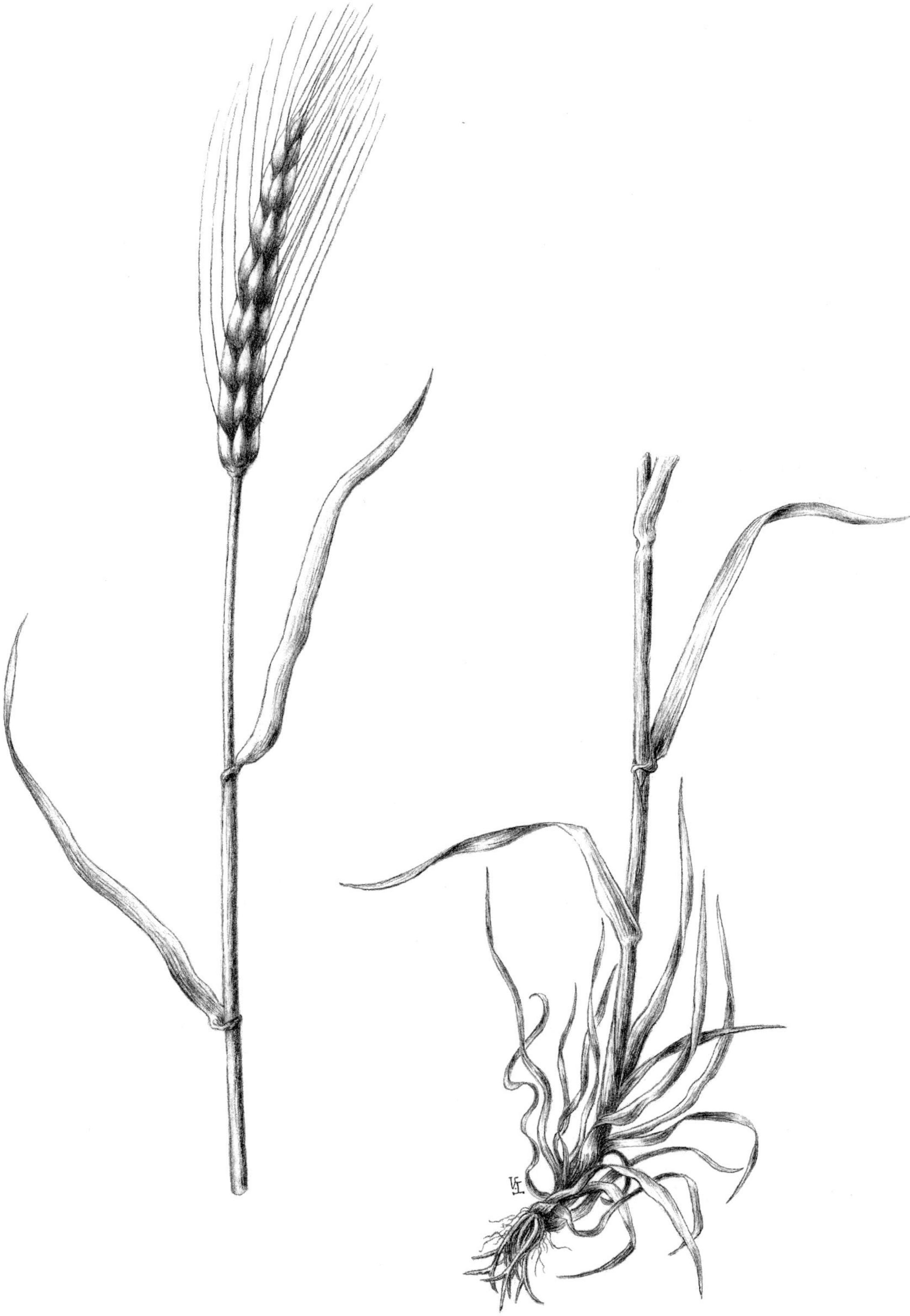

18 *Hypericum perforatum* L.

English, St. John's wort

Italian, *erba di San Giovanni*

St. John's wort, one of the lovely wild flowers growing amid the Pompeii excavations, is a perennial herb, twenty to sixty centimeters in height, having numerous slightly woody branched stems, and small leaves with numerous translucent dots, a feature that makes the species easy to recognize and is alluded to in its scientific name. The plant is distinguished by its delicate, deep yellow flowers with very small black dots on the margins (see Fig. 8). St. John's wort owes its name to the medieval belief that it protected against witchcraft, enchantment, and lightning, if gathered on St. John's (San Giovanni's) Day, June 24.

It is a medicinal plant much used at Pompeii. Boiled in water, it is a popular medicine: one glass of the liquid is believed to cleanse the system. The flowers, steeped in oil, are used for burns. In winter, around Christmas, the plant is used in cooking, especially for flavoring minestrone.

That *Hypericum perforatum*, the St. John's wort used by modern Pompeians, grew in the Vesuvian area in antiquity is evidenced by the flowering stems of this species found in the carbonized hay at Oplontis. It is this species that is still used for medicine throughout Italy.

Pliny has several references to *hypericon*, but it is difficult to identify the species that he refers to. He says *hypericon* has thin reddish stems a cubit high, and leaves like those of rue with pungent smell. It has black seeds in a pod, which check diarrhea and promote urine; taken with wine, it corrects bladder problems (*HN* 26.85). He lists many other ailments cured by *hypericon* (*HN* 26.86, 90, 117, 119, 129, 130, 158, 164), but none of the uses, except for treatment of burns, persists at Pompeii today. Pliny refers to another St. John's wort (*HN* 27.26,37) as "*androsaemon* or, as others have called it *ascyron*, which is not unlike *hypericon*." The smell is resinous, the leaves like those of rue, and when crushed it gives out a blood-colored juice. Besides treating burns, it is also used to cleanse the system, as in Pompeii today, and for sciatica, gout, and, since it staunches blood, for wounds.

Dioscorides' description (3.172) is similar. He says the plant *askyron* (ἄσκυρον), which some call "*androsimon* [man's blood] is a kind of *hyperikon*." It has small leaves, yellow flowers, fruit with the smell of resin, and when bruised yields a bloody juice. Popular fancy has always been struck by this blood-colored liquid which oozes from the peduncles when the flowers are pulled up. Dioscorides gives fewer medicinal uses: to cleanse the system, for sciatica, and for *ambusta* (burns).

Celsus gives only two medicinal uses of *hypericum*. The juice was used in making a lozenge to expel stones from the bladder (5.20.6). It was also one of the ingredients in the famous antidote King Mithridates was said to have taken daily to protect himself against poisoning (5.23.3). Galen recommends *hyperikon* as an emmenagogue and as a diuretic (*De simpl. med. temp. ac fac.* 8.20.5 = Kühn ed. 12:148).

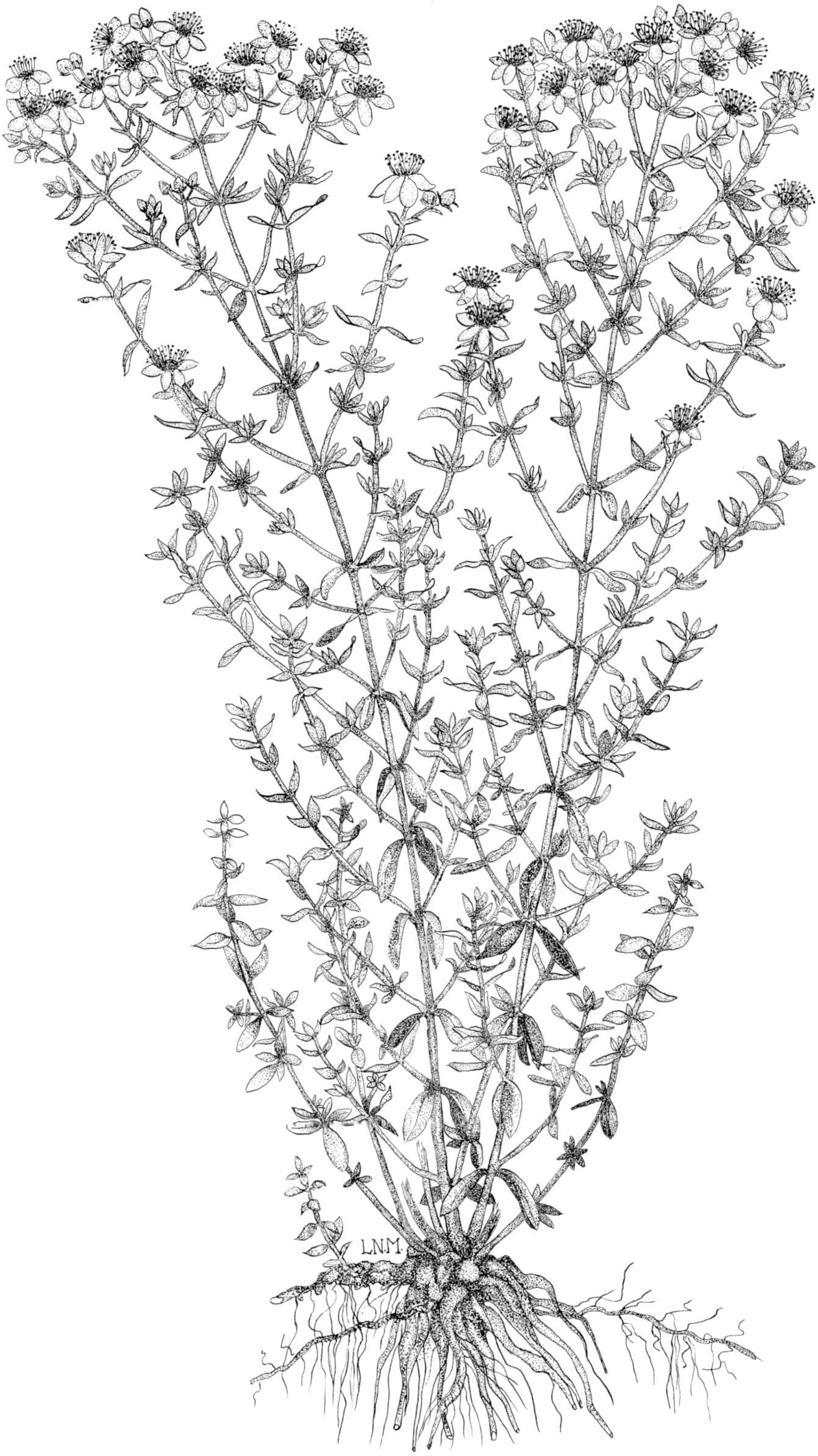
LNM.

19 *Juglans regia* L.

English, English or Persian walnut

Italian, *noce*

The stately walnut, which grows up to fifteen meters in height, is first mentioned by Theophrastus (3.14.4), who calls this tree the Persian nut (καρύα ἡ Περσίκη). *Juglans* was the classical Latin name for the walnut, a contraction from *Jovis glans,* the nut of Jupiter or Jove's acorns. Pliny (*HN* 15.87) says that the Greek name for the walnut proves that it "was sent to us from Persia by the kings, the best kind of walnut being called in Greek the 'Persian' and the 'Royal.'" Linnaeus uses as the scientific name *Juglans regia,* a combination of the Latin name with the adjective "royal."

Carbonized walnuts found in the excavations can be seen in the Naples Museum and at Herculaneum, and walnut shells were identified in the carbonized hay at Oplontis. Walnut pollen was identified in various gardens that I excavated.

The walnut is an important commercial crop at Pompeii today, and the nut highly favored, unlike the situation in antiquity. It has one important medicinal use today, as the basic ingredient used in making a very complicated tonic/medicine (*nocino, nocillo*) in which the Pompeians have great faith. I was given two different recipes and a bottle of the tonic, but I have never had the courage to try it. I was emphatically told that it was absolutely necessary to make both recipes on June 23, the day before San Giovanni's (St. John's) Day, June 24. I later learned that almost every family had its favorite recipe. Professor Ricciardi gave me his family recipe.

In antiquity the walnut was not greatly favored as a food. Pliny (*HN* 23.147) says that walnuts cause heaviness of the head. Even the trees and the leaves give out a poison that penetrates the brain. The kernels if eaten have the same effect, though the pain is less severe. He does say, however, that freshly gathered (and not yet dried) nuts are more agreeable. Apicius, who makes generous use of other nuts in his recipes, calls for walnuts only twice (6.5.3; 9.13.2). But the walnut was greatly esteemed for medicinal purposes. Oil made of walnuts, according to Pliny, is useful for mange and is injected into the ears for hardness of hearing, and an application relieves headache, but it is of a disagreeable taste (*HN* 23.88). He lists a great variety of uses: walnuts expel tapeworms, cure dysentery, can be applied to the bites of dogs and humans, and deaden the effects of poisons (*HN* 23.147–148). They were also used for dyeing wool, and the young nuts were a source of red hair-dye (*HN* 15.87).

Dioscorides (1.178), too, says the walnut, "the royal nut, which some call Persica," is harmful to the stomach and causes headaches, but he gives a long list of medicinal uses.

Scribonius includes walnuts in remedies for tumors, ulcers of the kidneys (143), bladder problems (148), and pain in the loins and palsy (156).

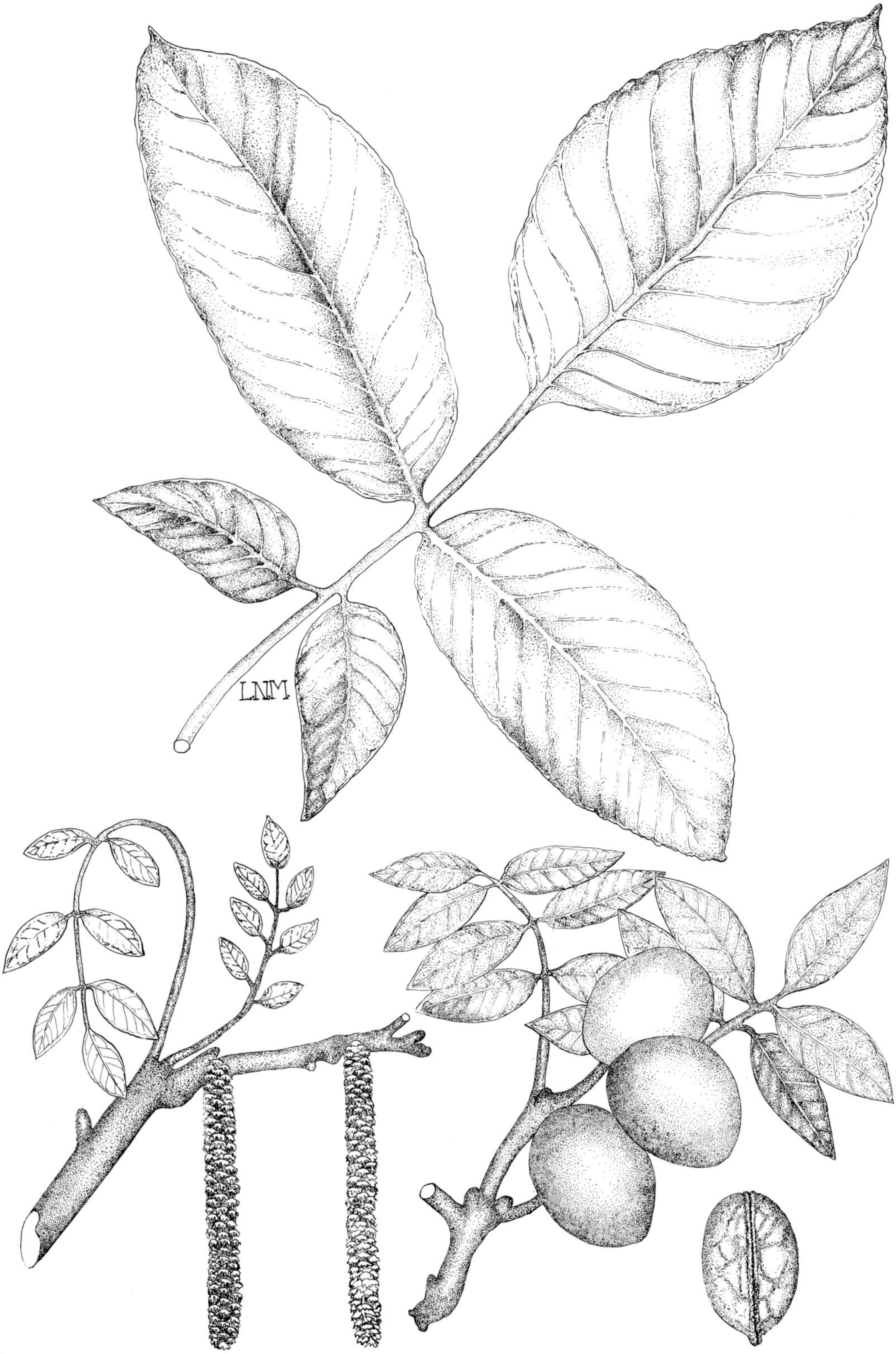
LNM

20 *Lactuca sativa* L.

English, lettuce

Italian, *lattuga*

The humble garden lettuce has long been cultivated in Europe. It is used today at Pompeii, as it was in antiquity, not only as food, but as a medicinal plant. Lettuce leaves are boiled in a little water and applied to swollen gums to cure the inflammation. Elsewhere in Italy a poultice of leaves is used for insomnia, and lettuce is used as a laxative and treatment for intestinal ailments, and for stomach problems in children.

Pliny has many references to *lactuca,* but he applies the name to many plants that are not lettuce. In the section on lettuce in his discussion of garden plants (*HN* 19.125–128), he says that all lettuces are believed to bring sleep. The emperor Augustus was cured by lettuce. Lettuce was also believed to increase the blood supply.

Theophrastus (7.2.4,9) describes lettuce (θρίδαξ) in his section on pot-herbs, but he gives no medicinal uses. Dioscorides (2.165) says that garden lettuce is good for the stomach and causes sleep. Too much, however, causes dullness of sight.

Columella (10.179–180), in his poetical description of the garden, speaks of lettuce "which can assuage sad loathing caused by lingering disease."

Celsus lists lettuce as a laxative (2.29.1), to produce sleep (for this purpose he recommends mostly the summer kinds in which the stalk is very milky [2.32]), and, dipped in vinegar, to soothe an aching spleen (4.16.2). The poet Martial (3.89) also speaks of lettuce as a laxative.

Scribonius uses lettuce in a prescription for stomach ailments (104) and in a purging pill (138). Galen, in his treatise *On Parts of the Body Affected,* says lettuce induces sleep (*De locis affectis* 2.5 = Kühn ed. 8:131).

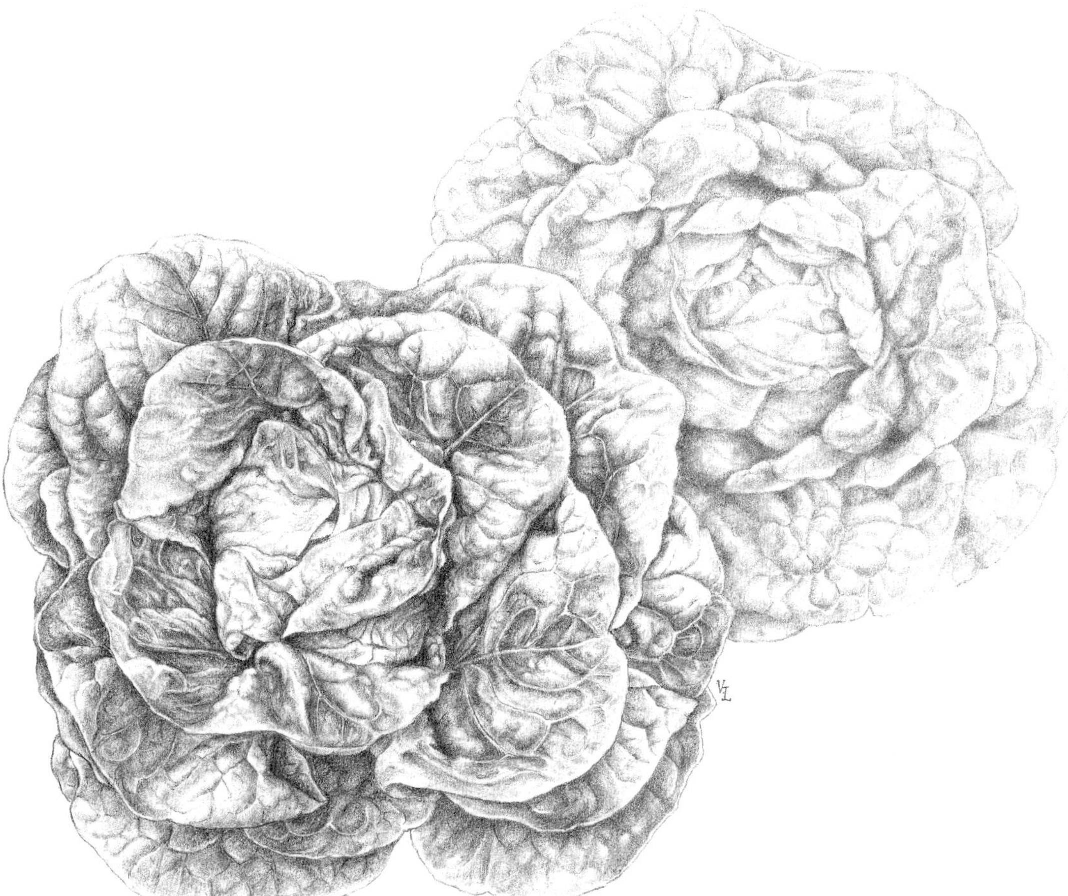

21 *Laurus nobilis* L.

English, laurel, bay tree

Italian, *alloro, lauro*

The beautiful laurel, with its glossy dark evergreen leaves and shining black berries, is native throughout the Mediterranean area, and also a favorite in ornamental gardens. The flowers, leaves, and berries, when crushed, are strongly aromatic. It grows as a bush or small tree two to ten meters in height. It was a delight to discover the road leading to the grotto of the Sibyl at Cumae lined with beautiful laurel trees.

The laurel was also used in ancient Pompeian gardens. In the early excavations in the rear peristyle garden of the House of the Faun, in front of the two lararia, archaeologists found the remains of a branch of laurel with the bones of a dove that had nested in it.

The laurel was much venerated in antiquity. Greek mythology tells how the beautiful maiden Daphne was loved by Apollo, but she would have none of him. When he pursued her, she prayed for help and was changed into the tree bearing her name. Thereupon the *daphne* (δάφνη) (Latin *laurus*) became the favorite tree of Apollo and sacred to him. The Roman poet Ovid (*Met.* 1.452–567) recounts the tale, and it is personified in stone in the famous statue of the baroque sculptor Bernini.

Pompeians today boil four or five leaves in a glass of water and drink the liquid for ailments of the liver, stomach, colon, and bowels, a treatment mild enough for children. For digestive problems they also use a mixture of boiled fennel seeds and chestnuts to which laurel is added or laurel leaves boiled with camomile.

Pliny gives a long list of medicinal uses (*HN* 23.152–158). Just like the present-day Pompeians, he recommends leaves boiled in water for bowel pains; berries for liver ailments. Dioscorides (1.106) gives a similar but shorter list of uses of the laurel. Soranus (1.65) lists it as an ingredient in one of the more gentle vaginal suppositories that causes an abortion. Celsus gives few medicinal uses of the laurel, most for external use, but says the berries were used internally for liver disease (4.15.3). Scribonius prescribes laurel berries for head ailments (3, 5) and in poultices for various ailments (262, 263).

Every good cook knows the value of the bay leaf. Apicius uses the berries as well as sprigs and shoots.

Victorious generals wore laurel crowns and carried laurel branches; their lictors bore fasces bound with laurel during a triumph. Pliny tells how an eagle dropped a white hen, holding in its beak a laurel branch with berries, from the sky into Livia's lap. The branch was planted and guarded with religious care. Thereafter, the emperor Augustus held a branch of the original tree and wore a wreath of its foliage in triumphs. Subsequent emperors did the same, and these branches were later planted—the origin of the famous laurel grove at Livia's villa at Prima Porta (*HN* 15.136–137). The ancestral images were decorated with laurel on special occasions (Cicero, *Pro Murena* 88). Laurel leaves were eaten to give an individual the power to prophesy. The custom of making a crown of laurel with berries for young scholars is the origin of the title *baccalaureate.*

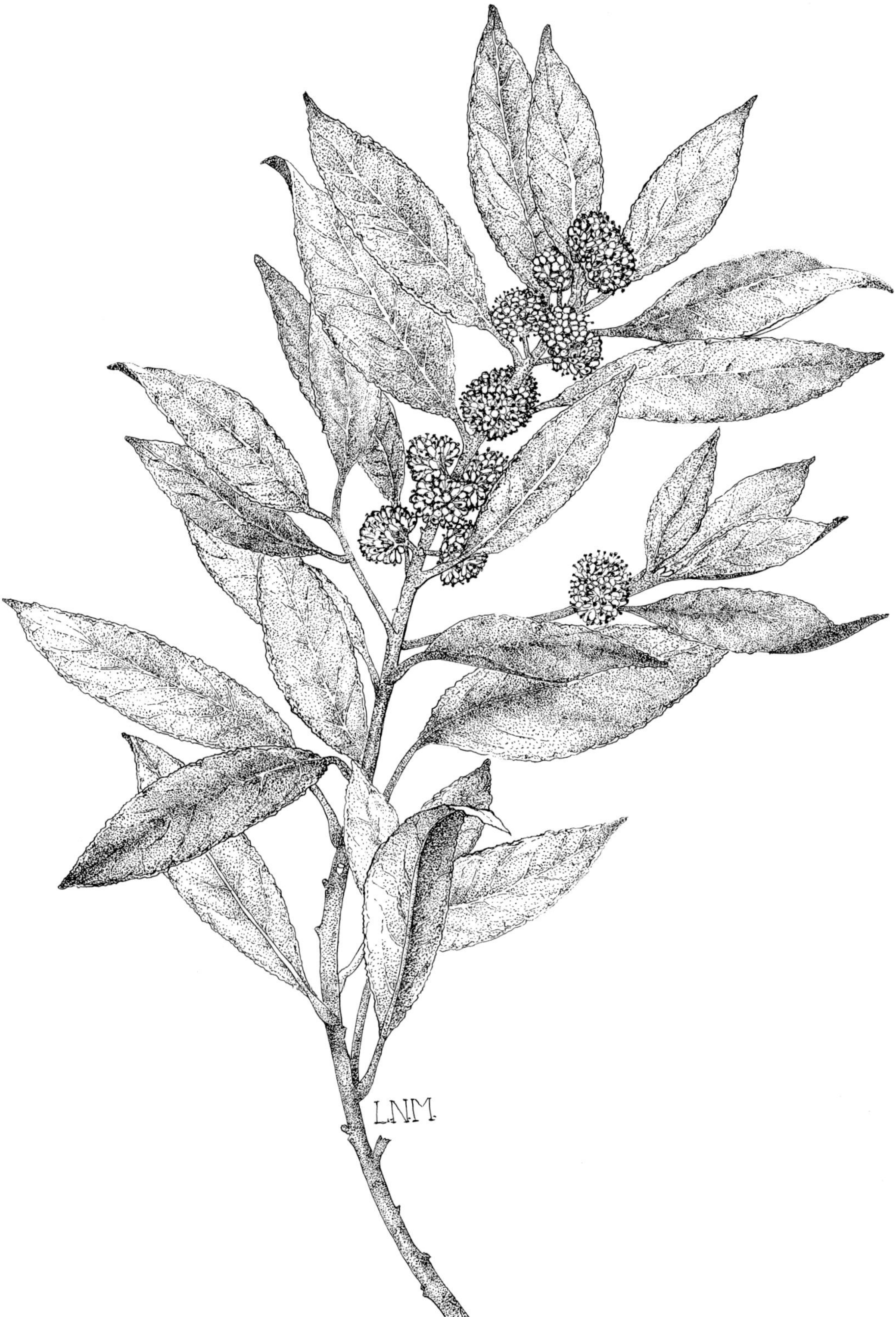
LNM

22 *Lobularia maritima* (L.) Desv. (*Alyssum maritimum* (L.) Lam.)

ENGLISH, SWEET ALYSSUM

Italian, *alisso*

This small perennial with close clusters of tiny sweet-scented flowers grows throughout the Mediterranean area. These white flowers growing in beautiful profusion in the excavated houses at Pompeii are an unforgettable sight.

My workmen told me that today they mix alyssum in a pan with oil or water, then fry or heat it as a compress or poultice for sore throat. Others told me that, fried in oil, it is applied to bruises on the arm or leg.

Sweet alyssum is indigenous to the Mediterranean area, but it is not mentioned in the preserved writings of any ancient author. However, many other plants that grew in antiquity (for example, many identified in the carbonized hay found at Oplontis) are not mentioned in our ancient sources, and no remains have been found of many plants that grew in antiquity.

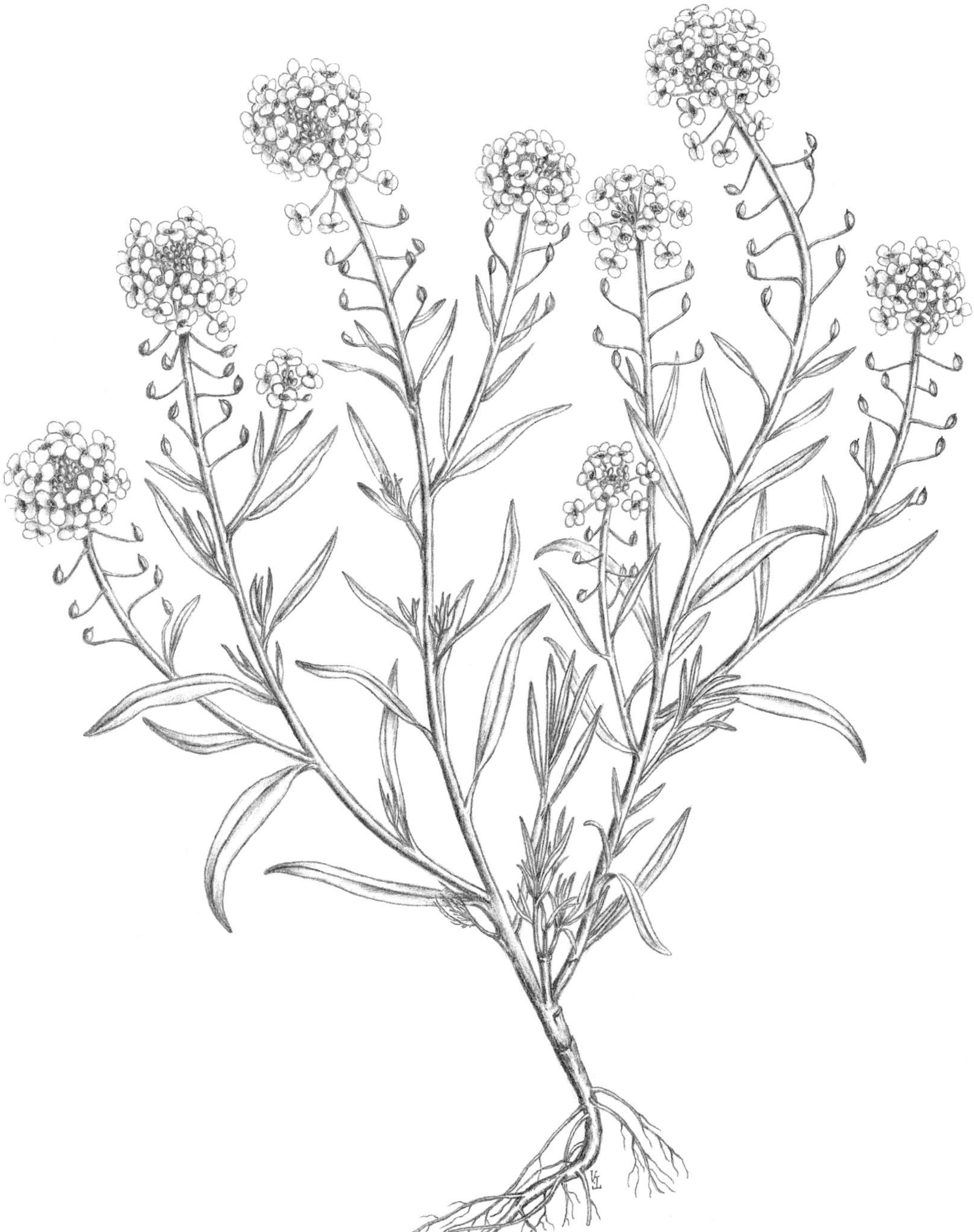

23 *Malus domestica* Borkh. (*Pyrus malus* L.)

English, apple

Italian, *melo*

The common apple, boiled together with the roots of mallow (*Malva sylvestris*), is used as a medicine at Pompeii for *bambini* with stomach problems. Apples boiled with hollyhock flowers are also used for children with stomach ailments. Elsewhere in Italy, the apple has more medicinal uses. The bark, gathered in the spring, the fruit, and sometimes the peelings are widely used in various infusions, syrups, and mixtures as a medicine.

The ancient Romans had many varieties of apples. We found a carbonized apple when excavating the rear garden of the villa of Poppaea at Oplontis.

According to Pliny (*NH* 23.104), certain "round" apples (*mala orbiculata*) arrested looseness of the bowels and vomiting and acted as a diuretic. Various sweet apples relaxed the stomach and bowels. He says that wild apples, which are like sour spring apples, arrest looseness of the bowels, and for this purpose they must be eaten unripe. According to Dioscorides (1.159) the leaves, blossoms, sprigs, and unripe fruit of all sorts of apple trees are binding. Celsus (4.26.5–6) prescribes apples for diarrhea.

Scribonius uses apples in a prescription (104) for stomach problems in which he calls for two varieties, "round" (*orbiculata*) and Scandian apples.

The gynecologist Soranus uses the apple in various prescriptions for treating women. He prescribes the external use of apples as a styptic remedy for upset stomach in pregnancy (1.50); an apple as "smelling salts" to revive a woman in labor (2.2); apples as food for a woman with hemorrhage of the uterus (3.41) or in difficult labor (4.7); and apples in a decoction for the flux (4.44), which was defined in antiquity as "an increased flow of blood through the uterus over a protracted period" (3.43).

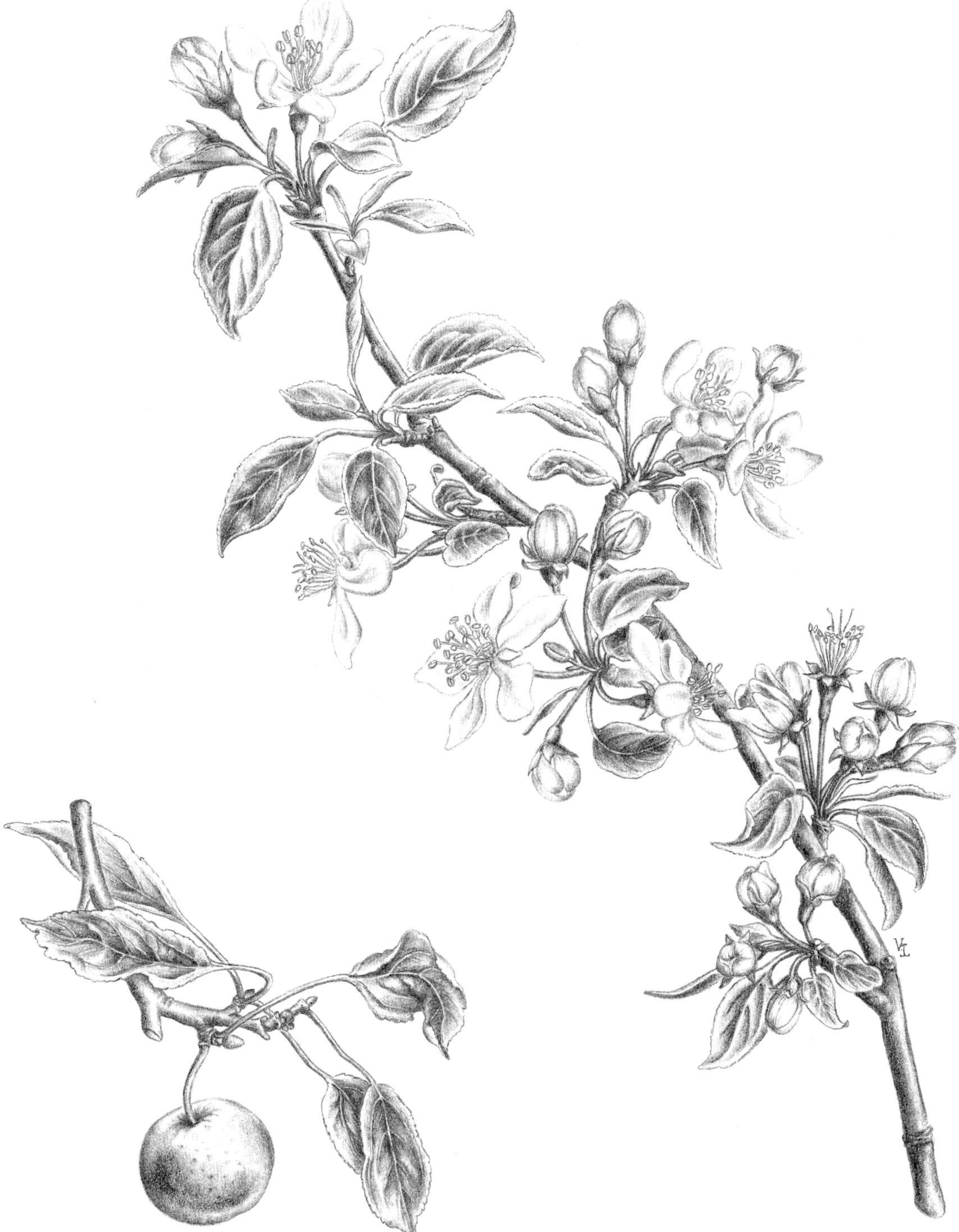

24 *Malva sylvestris* L.

English, common mallow

Italian, *malva*

The common mallow is a biennial or short-lived perennial, with broad round-lobed leaves and conspicuous rosy-violet flowers with darker stripes. The flowers are in stalked clusters in the axils of the leaves. The plant grows 30 to 150 centimeters high. Branches bearing the leaves and fruit of common mallow were found in the carbonized hay at Oplontis. Mallow pollen was also found (see Fig. 22).

At Pompeii today, the root and leaves of common mallow are washed, boiled together, and used for toothache and for stomach problems; this liquid is also highly regarded as a cough medicine. The leaves alone boiled in water are used for toothache, the roots alone boiled in water for stomach problems, or for children with stomach problems, boiled with apple (see above, no. 23). Mallow roots are also boiled with roots of knotgrass and rhizomes of Bermuda grass for stomach problems.

In antiquity the mallow was also used for toothache and as a cough medicine. The root of a single stem was put around an aching tooth until the pain ceased (Pliny *HN* 20.224). The root boiled in milk and taken as a broth relieved a cough in five days (*HN* 20.225). In addition to the ailments for which it is used today, Pliny gives many, many more medicinal uses of the mallow (*malva*) (*HN* 20.222–230) and adds that it is an aphrodisiac. It is difficult to know just what species of mallow the ancient authors are referring to, but as we have seen, *Malva sylvestris,* which is used at Pompeii today, also grew in the area in antiquity. Pliny says that the most wonderful thing is that anyone who swallows daily half a cyathus (4 teaspoons) of mallow juice will be immune to all diseases! The cyathus was a small ladle used for transferring wine from the mixing bowl to the drinking cup.

Dioscorides (2.144), in his discussion of the mallow (μαλάχη), may be discussing both the common mallow and the hollyhock in the same passage (see above, no. 2). Celsus prescribes a decoction of mallow for a soothing enema (2.12.1.D–E). Scribonius uses the mallow in a medicine for the eyes, and for headaches (99); mallow seeds in a medicine for bladder problems (147); and in medicines for various other ills (184, 186).

The ancient Romans also made much use of the common mallow as food. Apicius gives various recipes for its use: as a vegetable (3,8; 4,2.10), in barley soup (4.4.2), and in a stuffing for suckling-pig (88.7.14).

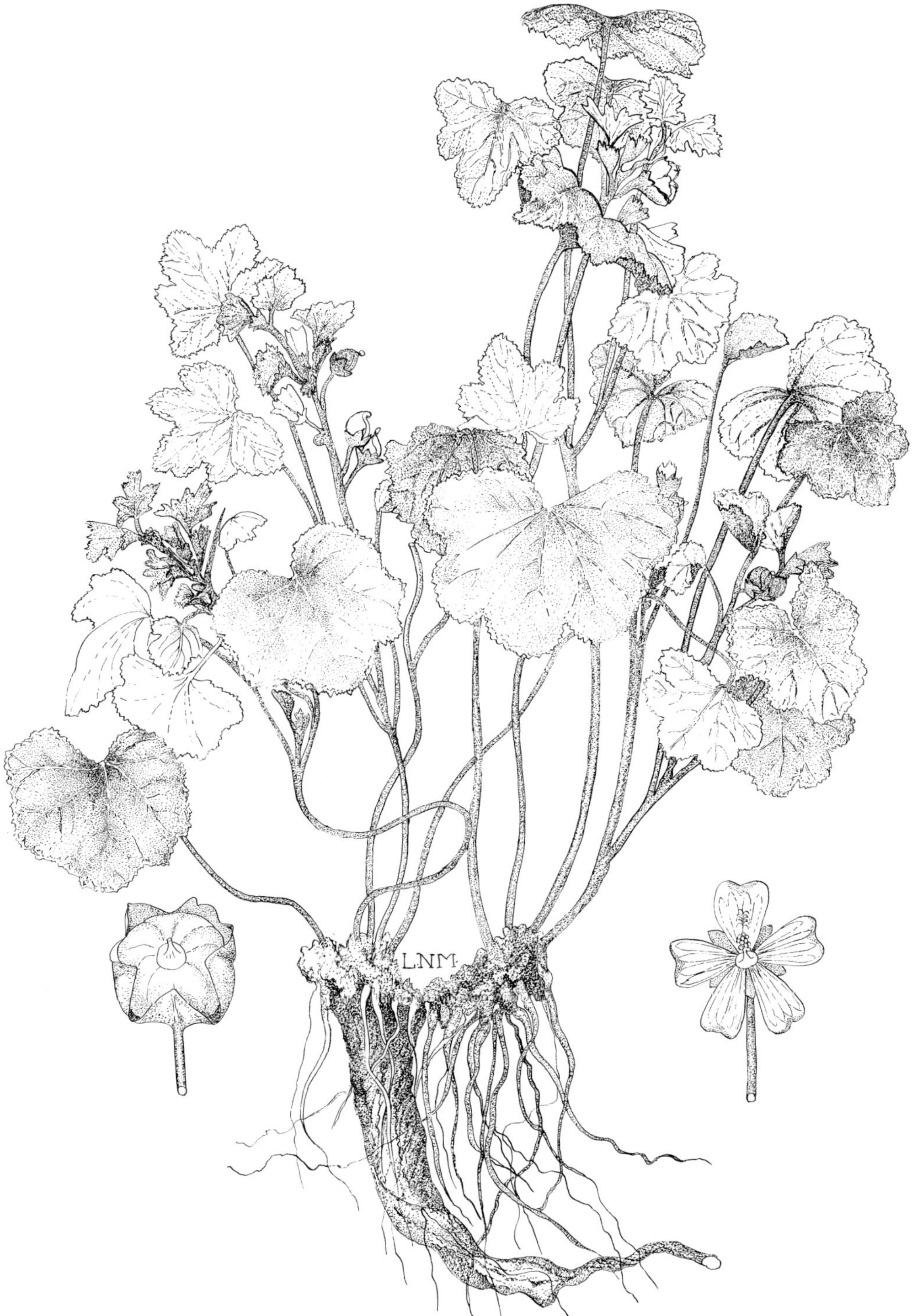
LNM

25 *Mentha suaveolens* Ehrh.

English, apple mint

Italian, *menta selvatica*

This mint, a perennial forty to one hundred centimeters in height, with white hairy stems and whitish or pink flowers, has a sickly sweet scent.

According to myth, mint (*menta*) got its name from the nymph Menthe or Mintha, the mistress of Hades, god of the underworld. She was trampled underfoot by his queen Persephone; she then became the plant named after her, which some call "sweet-scented" (ἡδύοσμον) because it smells the sweeter when trodden upon (Strabo, *Geography* 8.3.14). Pliny tells us:

> The name of mint has been altered in Greece because of its sweet scent; it used to be called *mintha,* from which our ancestors derived the Latin name, but now it has begun to be called by a Greek word meaning "sweet-scented." It is agreeable for stuffing cushions, and pervades the tables with its scent at country banquets. (*HN* 19.159–160)

This mint was recommended to me by the present-day Pompeians for kidney problems. They also assured me that chewing three leaves would take care of stomach problems.

It is very difficult to identify what mint is prescribed by the ancient authors as a specific for a particular ailment (see above, no. 4). Pliny (*HN* 20.151) does say that "a three-finger pinch of dried mint (*menta*) taken in water relieves stomach ache."

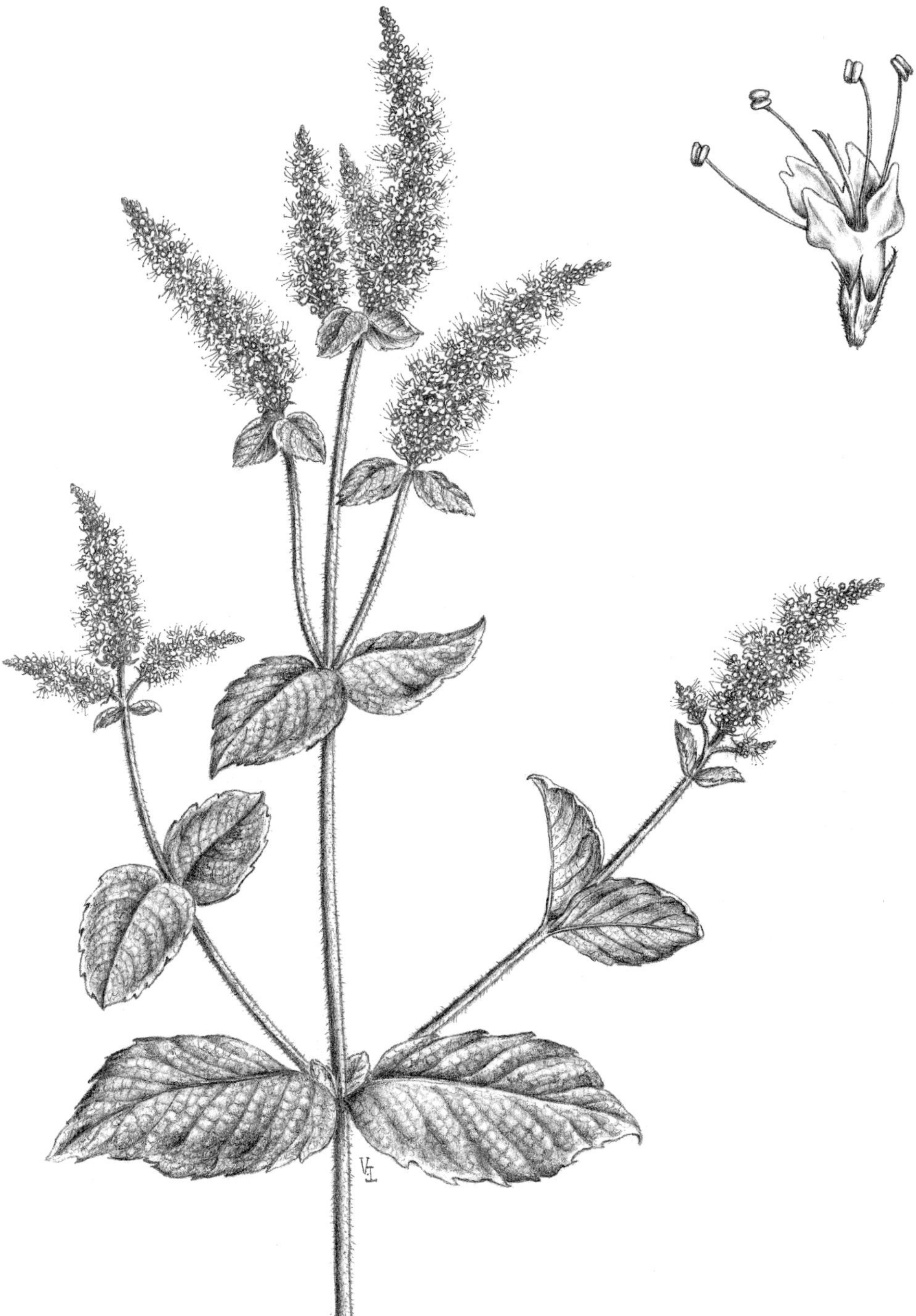

26 *Myrtus communis* L.

English, myrtle

Italian, *mirto, mortella*

This beautiful evergreen shrub (sometimes a small tree) with small shining dark green leaves, sweet-scented lacy white flowers, and blue-black berries, was appropriately esteemed at Pompeii in antiquity as the symbol of love; it was sacred to Venus, the patron deity of the ancient city.

The poet Ovid tells us that the myrtle (*myrtus*) protected Venus in a time of great need:

> Naked, she was drying on the shore her oozy locks, when the satyrs, a wanton crew, espied the goddess. She perceived it, and screened her body by myrtle interposed: that done, she was safe. (*Fasti* 141–144)

At Pompeii, a tonic, which I was told was very good for the stomach, has as its basic ingredient one cup of myrtle berries, to which is added three hundred grams of sugar, five hundred to six hundred grams of water, and various flavorings. The large bowl of myrtle berries found in the excavations may have been gathered for use as medicine, or perhaps for cooking.

Cato, in his treatise *On Agriculture* (*De re rustica* 125), gives a recipe for myrtle wine which he says "is a remedy for indigestion, for pain in the side, and for colic." Both Pliny and Dioscorides (μυρσίνη) recognize the value of the myrtle berry for stomach ailments. They recommend, among many other medicinal uses, both myrtle berries and leaves for everything from stomach, eye, heart, bladder, and bowel problems, to hair loss, freckles, and hangnails (Pliny, *HN* 15.124, 23.87,159–165; Dioscorides 1.155). Celsus gives various external uses of myrtle, including myrtle oil in soothing plasters for eczema of the scalp (6.2.2).

Soranus gives a number of uses of the myrtle for infants and small children. Leaves put in the cradle give it a sweet smell (2.16); for skin afflictions he prescribes a warm decoction using myrtle, and for more severe skin ulcers, an ointment of myrtle oil (2.52). Soranus also uses myrtle as an ingredient in various contraceptives and abortifacients (1.61,63,65).

The myrtle berry was a source of both wine and oil (Columella 12.38; Pliny, *HN* 15.118,123). Pliny says that the myrtle berry played the role of pepper before black pepper was known in Italy. He goes on to say that it was still used in making myrtle sausage and that the flavor of wild boar was improved by using myrtle berries (*HN* 15.118). Apicius frequently uses myrtle berries in his recipes.

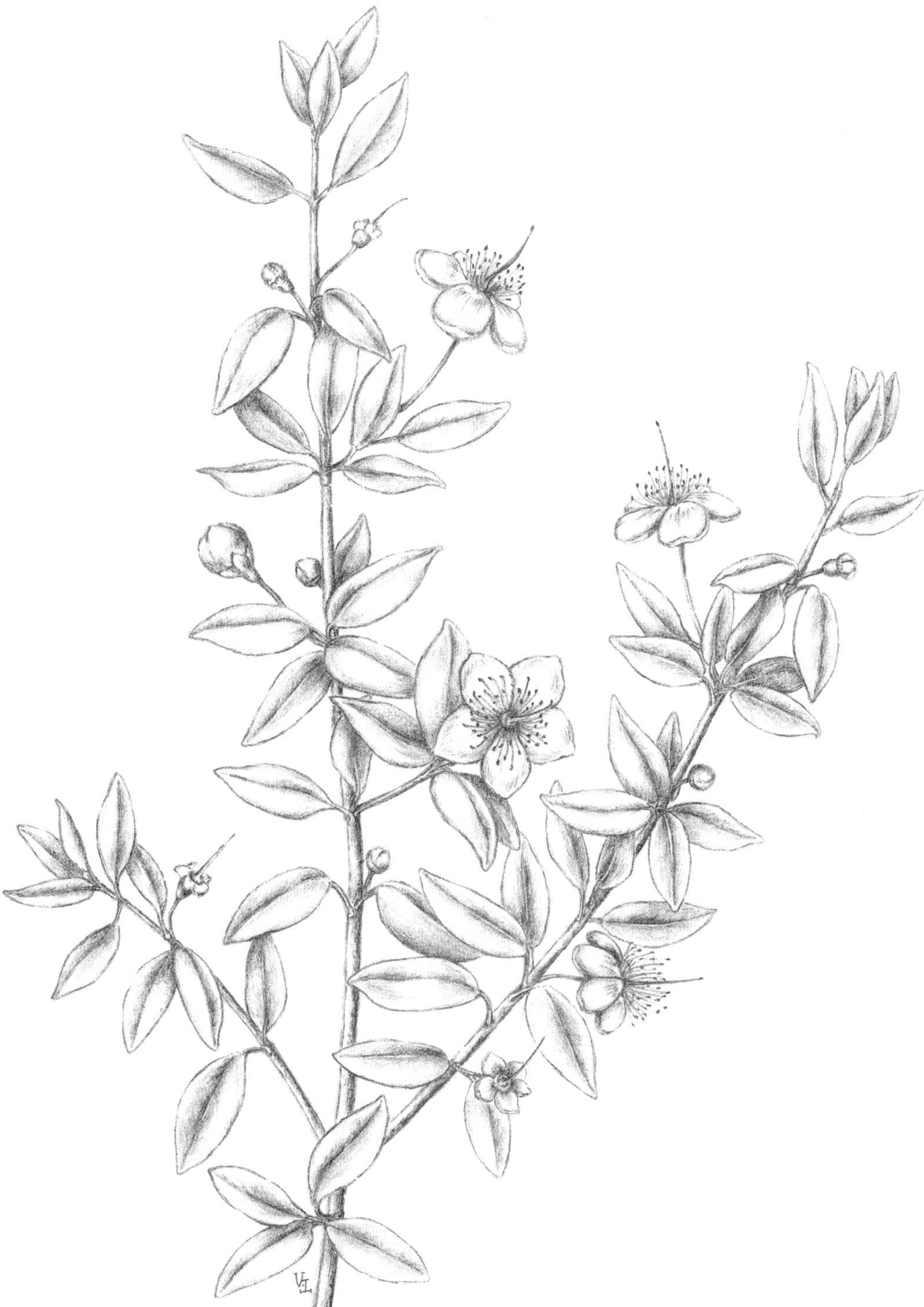

27 *Parietaria officinalis* L.

ENGLISH, WALL PELLITORY

Italian, *erba muraiola vetriola*

Another medicinal plant strongly recommended by the women who lived within the shadow of the ancient city was a plant that hangs in clumps from the walls of the amphitheater at Pompeii, as well as elsewhere on walls throughout the excavations. They knew it only as the *erba di muro* (the wall herb), a perfectly good Italian name, and they told me that it was an excellent cure when crushed and applied directly to bruises and sprains. To illustrate, one of the women lifted her skirt and showed me where she had that day applied it to a bad bruise on her thigh. She knew from experience that the bruise would soon be healed. I didn't recognize the plant, but Dr. Meyer identified the specimen that she gave me as wall pellitory (*Parietaria officinalis* L.), a close relative of another wall pellitory (*P. diffusa* Mert. & Koch), which also grows in the excavations. Both belong to the nettle family. The herb is steeped in water, but not boiled, and the liquid is drunk for stomach ailments.

This plant was also highly regarded by the ancient Greeks and Romans. Celsus (2.33.2) refers to this plant as *herba muralis,* the Latin equivalent of the present-day Italian name. The ancient Romans also knew the plant as *herba parietaria* (the herb belonging to the walls). According to the Roman historian Aurelius Victor (*Epitome de Caesaribus* 41), the emperor Constantine gave the emperor Trajan the nickname of *herba parietaria* because of the many inscriptions he had placed on the buildings he erected.

Both Pliny (*NH* 21.176; 22.43–44), who calls it *parthenium,* and Dioscorides (4.86), who calls it *elxine* (ἐλξίνη), list a variety of medicinal uses for this plant, but it was with mounting excitement that I read in Pliny that this plant was prescribed by the Greek goddess Athena to heal severe bruises. She appeared to Pericles in a dream, telling him to use this plant to cure his favorite slave who had fallen from the roof while working on the Parthenon (on the Propylaea, according to Plutarch, *Pericles* 13.7–8). The slave was cured, and the plant was henceforth called *parthenium,* after Athena Parthenos, and was consecrated to this goddess.

Celsus recommends the use of *herba muralis,* which he says the Greeks called *parthenion* (2.33.2), for external use, including painful joints (4.31.7).

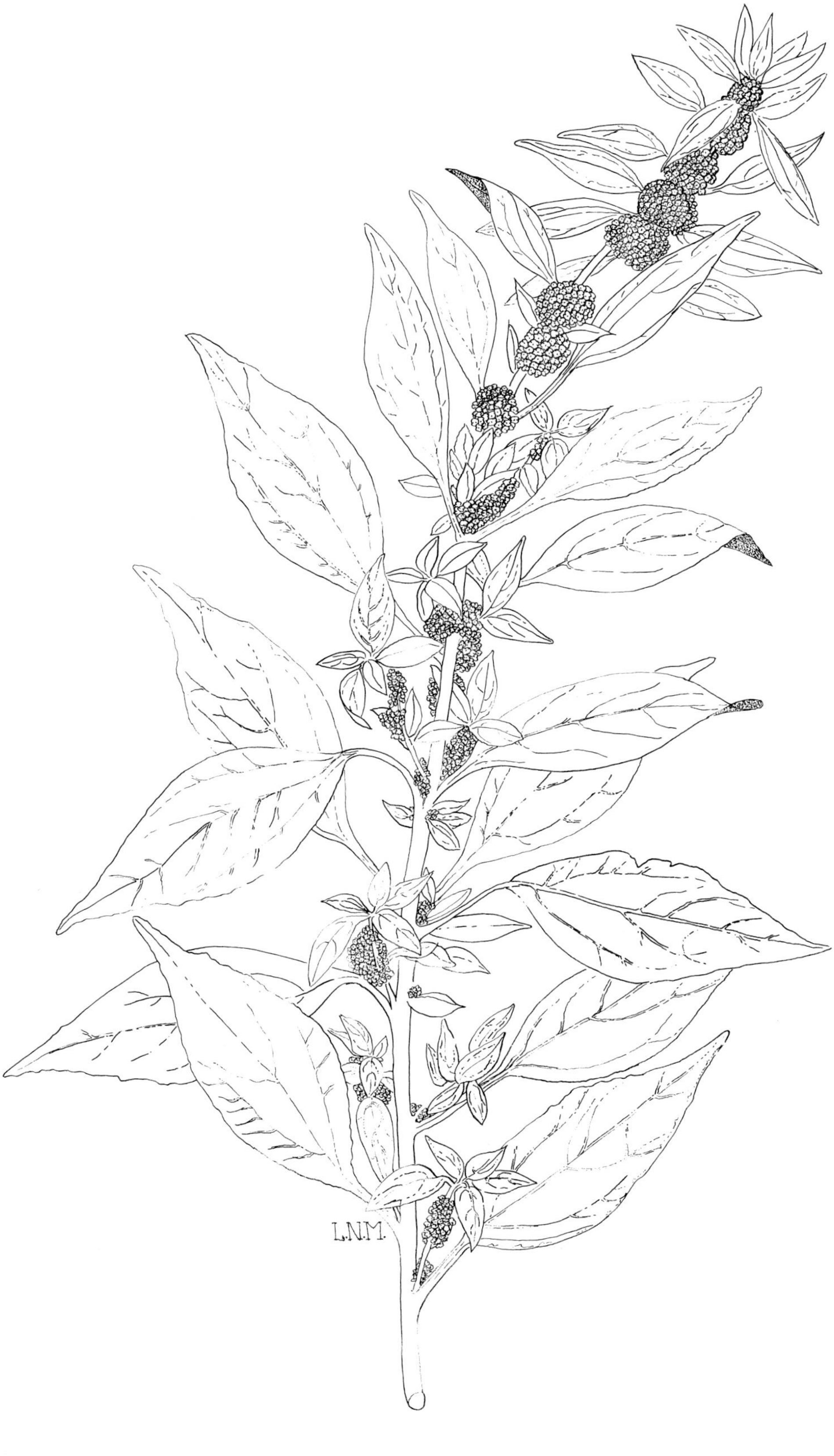
L.N.M.

28 *Petroselinum crispum* (Miller) A. W. Hill (*P. sativum* Hoffm.)

ENGLISH, PARSLEY

Italian, *prezzemolo*

At Pompeii they told me that parsley leaves shaped into a suppository and inserted into the vagina would cause an abortion. A suppository of parsley leaves is also inserted into the rectum of babies and children, if constipated, to stimulate an evacuation. These uses, among many, are also reported in the area of Rome (Guarrera, p. 159).

Pliny (*HN* 20.114) warns against using parsley because he says that it causes sterility. But he is, in fact, furnishing information that it is a contraceptive. The word he uses for parsley in this passage is *apium.* The Romans used this name (which in some contexts means "celery") as well as *petroselinum* for parsley. In another passage Pliny (*HN* 20.118) says that parsley (*petroselinum*) is especially good for abscesses. Dioscorides (3.76) lists parsley (ὀρειοσέλινον) as an emmenagogue, also for pain in the side, and for stomach, kidney, and bladder problems.

Scribonius gives eight prescriptions that contain parsley (106, 120, 126, 144, 145, 152, 176, 177) — more than for any other medicinal plant used at Pompeii, except rue. These are prescribed for a variety of ailments, including the use of parsley as an emmenagogue (106). Riddle (*Contraception and Abortion* pp. 84–85) points out that Scribonius was opposed to abortion, but that he "doubtless did not know that he delivered practical information about the procedure when he discussed emmenagogues."

Celsus uses the word *apium* to refer to both celery (*Apium graveolens* L.) and parsley (*Petroselinum crispum*), which he lists as a diuretic (2.31) and for other internal uses. Galen, in his treatise *On Remedies,* lists parsley as one of the plants in a prescription for an abortifacient that would expel a fetus without pain (*De antidotis* 2.1 = Kühn ed. 14:114–115).

Apicius (1.13) includes parsley in a medicine that aids digestion, prevents colds, and works as a laxative.

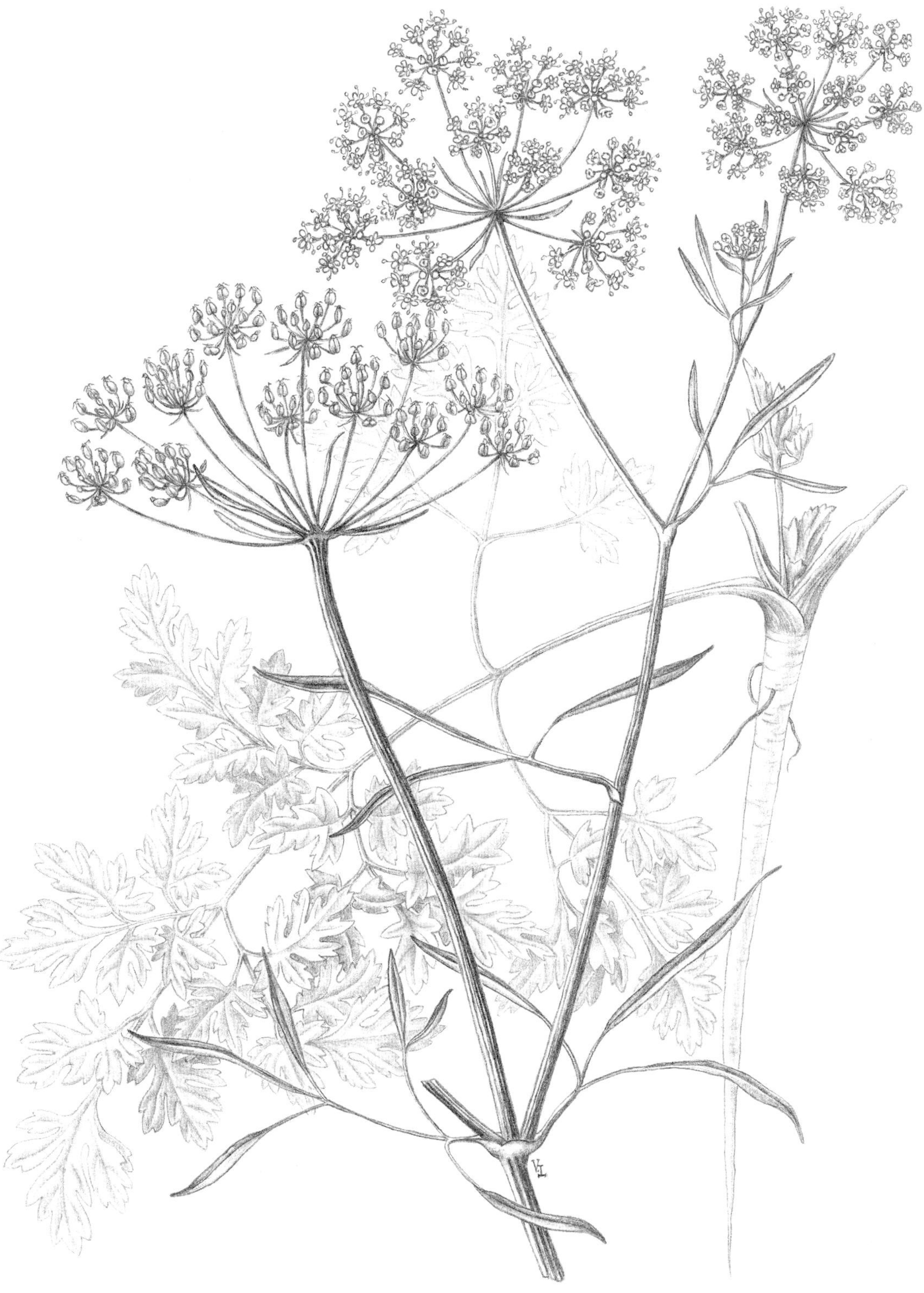

29 *Plantago major* L.

English, plantain

Italian, *piantaggine, piantaggine maggiore*

This common weed is a very attractive little plant, an herbaceous perennial, with large, elliptic leaves arranged in a rosette, and with scapes of minute greenish flowers (see Fig. 5). We know that this weed also infested the ancient gardens, for its pollen has been identified in my excavations.

At Pompeii today, to treat colitis, five leaves are heated in one-half to one-fourth liter of water and the liquid drunk, when cool, every other day.

Plantain had a multitude of medicinal uses in antiquity which are listed in great detail by both Pliny (*plantago*) and Dioscorides. Both authors (Dioscorides 2.153; Pliny, *HN* 25.80) distinguish between two kinds of plantain: the smaller, with narrower and darker leaves (*Plantago lagopus* L.), and the larger, with broader leaves (*Plantago major* L.). Both plants have the same medicinal properties. Theophrastus (7.10.3) and Dioscorides, who says that it flowers on a stalk, refer to plantain as *arnoglosson* (ἀρνόγλωσσον), or "lamb's tongue," a common name for the weed today. Celsus prescribes plantain for various ailments, including dysentery (4.23.2).

Scribonius includes plantain in prescriptions for eye salve (21, 31) and to treat eruptions of blood (83, 86). Soranus also lists a variety of uses, including a poultice for skin ulcers for infants (2.52), and, for infant diarrhea, the injection of a cyathus of the juice of plantain by means of a small ear syringe (2.56).

Pliny, in speaking of the dishonesty of herbalists, says they keep back part of some plants, such as plantain: "If they think their pay insufficient and look for further employment, they bury in the same place [in which they found it] the part they kept back, I suppose to make the complaints they have cured break out again" (*HN* 21.144).

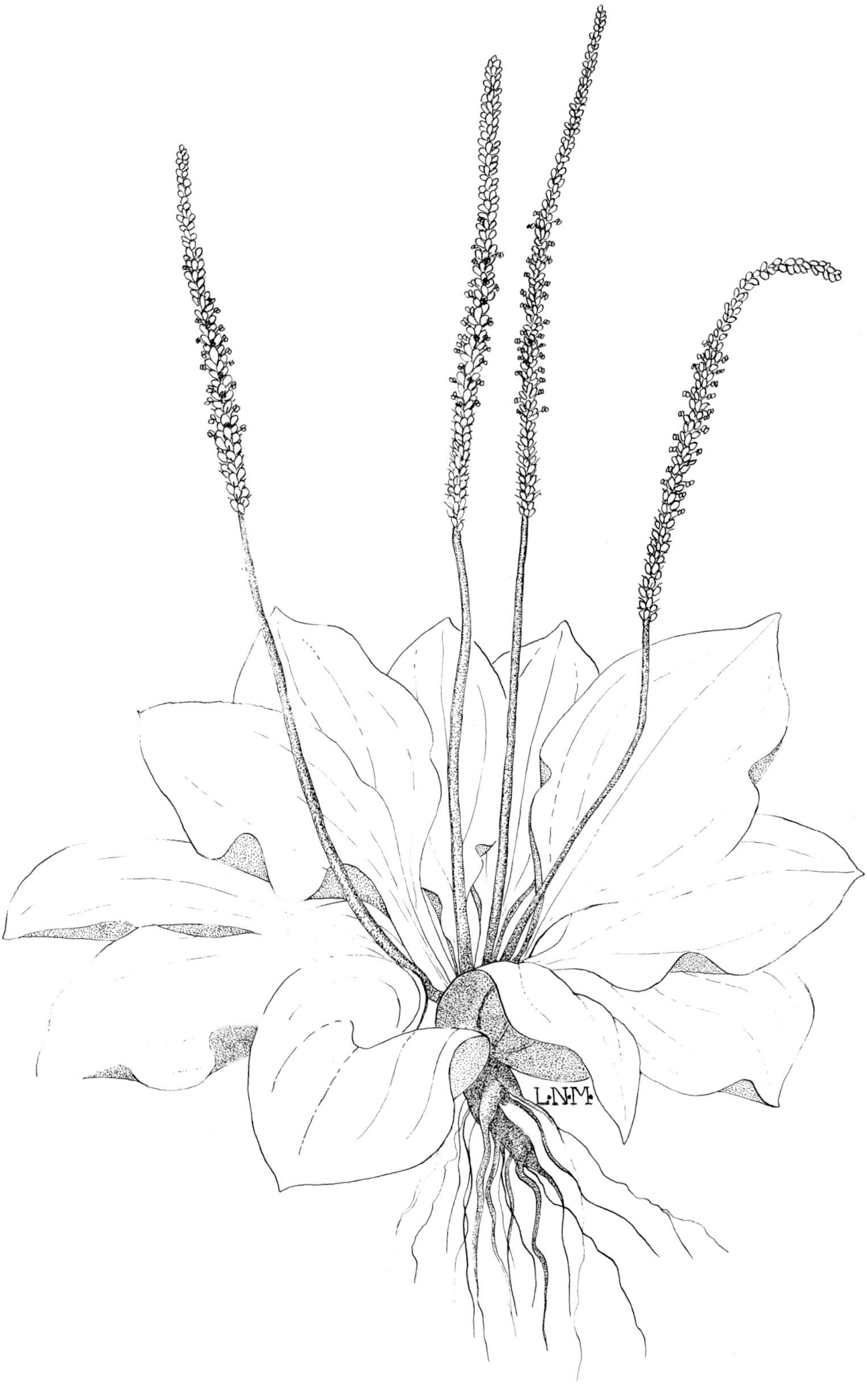
LNM

30 *Polygonum aviculare* L.

English, knotgrass

Italian, *centinodia, correggiola*

Knotgrass was the only herb that I found used at Pompeii for heart trouble. It is boiled in water, and the liquid drunk. Heart trouble is not one of the major health problems of the Italians, with their low-cholesterol, unsaturated-fat diet. Knotgrass is boiled in water with tender blackberry tips, fennel, and Bermuda grass, and sweetened with sugar; the hot liquid is drunk for colds, the cold liquid for digestive problems. The roots of knotgrass are boiled in water with the rhizomes of Bermuda grass and the common mallow and the infusion used for stomach ailments. The Pompeians today refer to this plant as *centinodia* (one hundred knots).

This weed invaded the farmland at the *villa rustica* in the *località villa Regina* that I excavated at Boscoreale near Pompeii, for its pollen has been identified in the excavations.

It was a popular medicine in antiquity. Pliny lists many conditions treated with knotgrass, including digestive ailments and colds (*HN* 27.114–117), as at Pompeii today. He says that the Greeks called this plant *polygonum,* the Romans *sanguinaria* (*HN* 27.113). He then adds that its juice, taken with wine, stops hemorrhage in any part of the body and the spitting of blood. In another passage (*HN* 26.158) he says that *polygonum* taken in drink purges the uterus. The agricultural writer Columella (6.12.5), in discussing the treatment of oxen, says that "incisions made with the knife can also be treated, as Cornelius Celsus taught, by means of . . . the staunching plant (*sanguinalis herba*), which the Greeks call *polygonum.*" Celsus speaks of the ability of this plant, which he calls *herba sanguinalis,* to stop bleeding (5.1). Its juice is very rich in tannin and gallic acid, which makes it a powerful astringent, able to stop hemorrhaging. Soranus (3.41) treats hemorrhage of the uterus with a plaster of knotgrass or an injection of knotgrass juice. The plant is known to present-day Italians as *sanguinaria,* because it staunches blood. Scribonius also prescribes knotgrass for hemorrhaging, and for several other purposes (2, 83, 93). He uses knotgrass (*polygonion*) in prescriptions for head problems (2), eruptions of blood from the arteries, lungs, or heart (83), and as an antidote (193). Pliny says no other plant is kept more in a dry state. Dioscorides (4.4) describes knotgrass (πολύγονον) as a tender plant with joints, creeping on the earth like grass. He also gives it as a specific for many ailments.

Linnaeus used *polygonum* as the generic name of the plant.

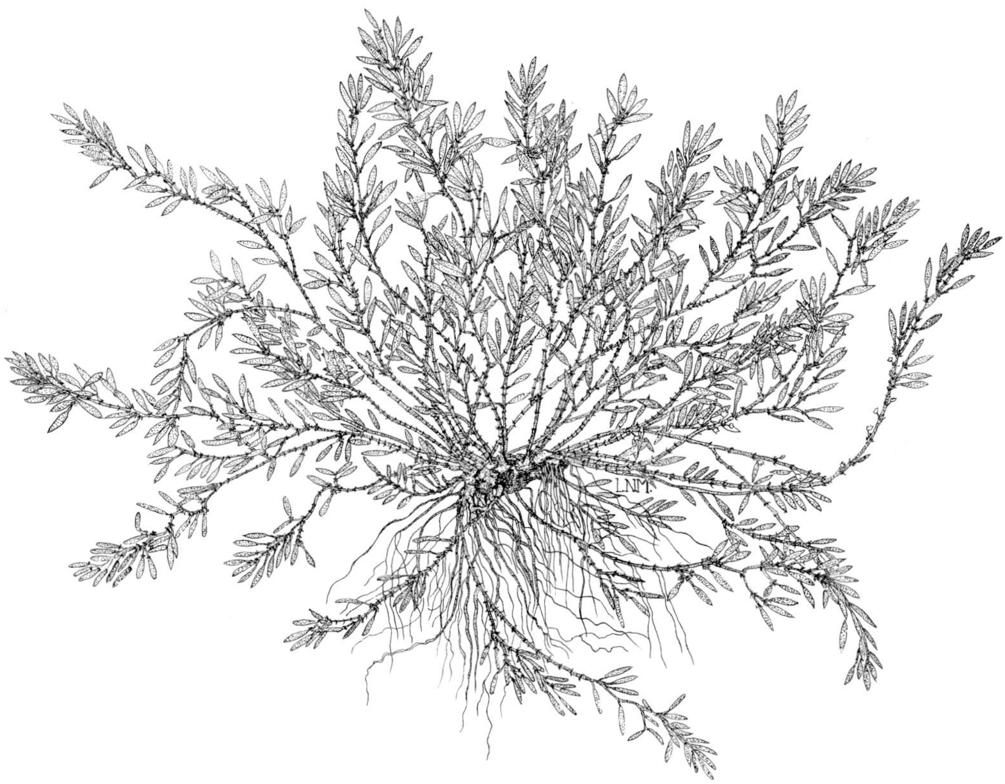
LNM

31 *Portulaca oleracea* L.

English, purslane

Italian, *portulaca, porcellana*

Purslane is a pesky, low-growing, annual garden weed, with tiny yellow flowers, that spreads widely in loose mats. But its dark green, juicy, succulent leaves are valued at Pompeii as a diuretic. Today the Pompeians use purslane as a salad plant and as a cooked vegetable, similar to spinach. Because of its drought-resistant qualities, it is prized in Greece as a salad vegetable, for it is available even in the dry season.

It was also used for food by the ancient Romans, and Columella (12.13.2) gives directions for preserving purslane (*portulaca*) by pickling it.

Pliny (*HN* 13.120) is probably referring to purslane when he erroneously speaks of *andrachle* (*andrachne*). He too says that it is gathered for food, that it is cooling and astringent, and good for eye problems, earache, and headaches (*HN* 25.162). Dioscorides (2.150–151) calls purslane *andrachne* (ἀνδράχνη). Scribonius has two prescriptions that include purslane (*portulaca*), for teeth problems (53) and gout (158). Soranus uses purslane as a poultice for skin ulcers in infants (2.52), and for plasters in hemorrhage of the uterus (3.41).

Celsus (2.20.1), like the modern Pompeians, recommends purslane as a food, as a diuretic (4.16.3), and chewed to check bleeding of the gums (4.11.5). Galen, however, in his treatise *On the Properties of Foods,* says purslane is of little value as a food (*De alimentorum facultatibus* 2.46 = Kühn ed. 6:46 = *CMG* 5.4.2:314).

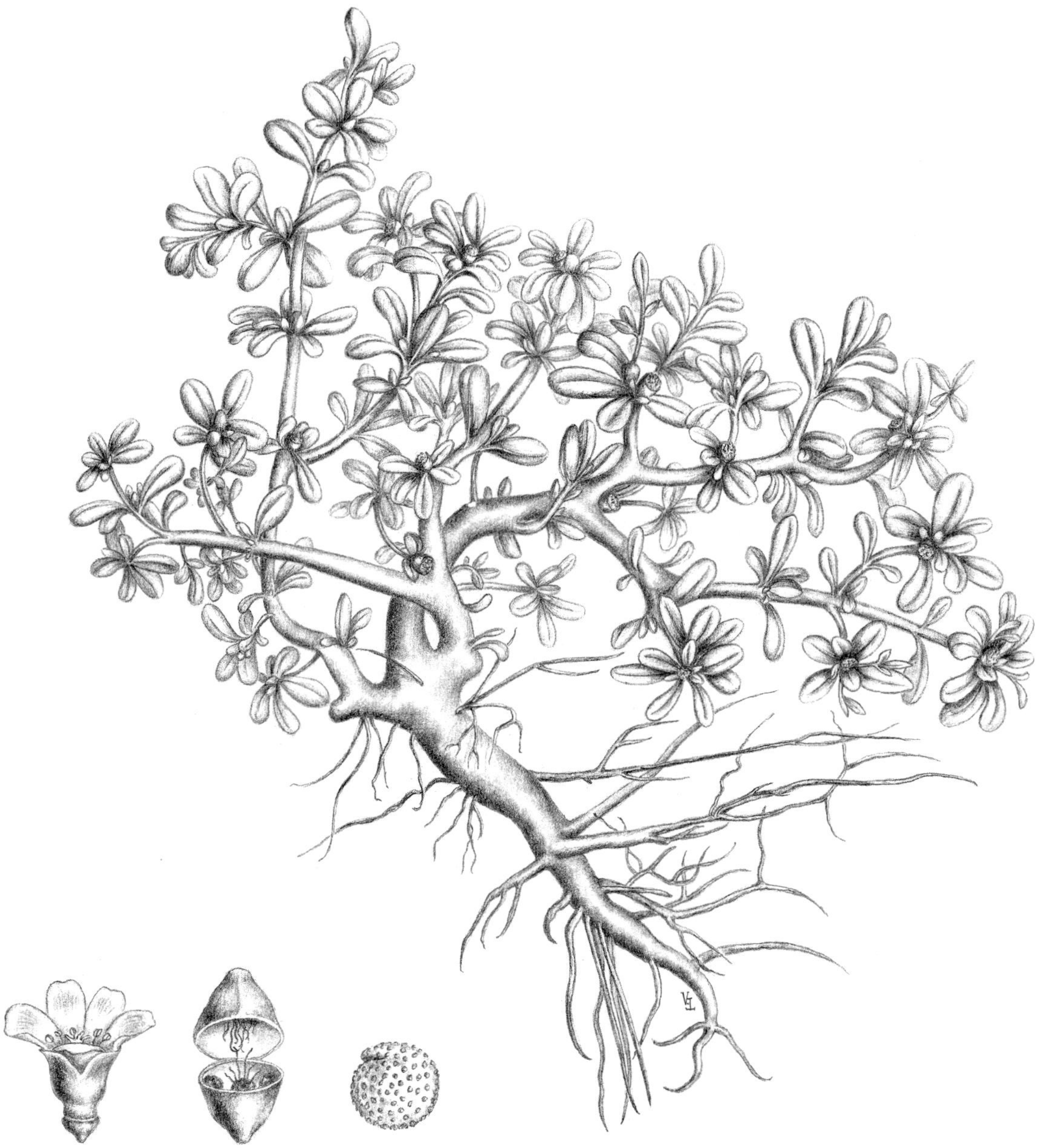

32 *Rubus ulmifolius* Schott

English, bramble, wild blackberry

Italian, *rovo, more di rovo*

Brambles are the scourge of the excavations today, for if left unchecked they completely take over an excavated site. Even so, I found their fruit was eagerly sought by my workmen, who were prone to leave a vine here and there for future picking. The ever-present bramble was found in the carbonized hay at Oplontis.

Women living in the excavations spoke highly of a medicine made by boiling the tender tips of brambles in water, along with knotgrass, Bermuda grass, and fennel. With sugar added, it was drunk hot for colds, and cold to aid digestion.

The bramble was also a pest in antiquity. But Pliny writes, "Not even brambles did Nature create for harmful purposes only, and so she has given them their black berries, that are food even for men" (*HN* 24.117). The Roman poet Ovid (*Met.* 1.105) speaks of the "berries hanging thick upon the prickly bramble." Pliny comments on another value of the bramble:

> Nature has likewise also taught the art of reproducing from layers. Brambles curving over with their slender and also excessively long shoots plant their ends in the earth again and sprout afresh out of themselves, in a manner that would fill up the whole place if resistance were not offered by cultivation. . . .
>
> Thus a most evil and execrable circumstance has nevertheless taught the use of the layer and the quickset. (*HN* 17.96)

Pliny (*HN* 16.176) gives still another use of the bramble: after the thorns are cut off, they serve as ties for grapevines.

The medicinal uses of the bramble were almost infinite in antiquity (Pliny, *HN* 24.117–120: *rubus;* Dioscorides 4.37: βάτος). Almost all parts of the plant—the tender shoots, leaves, the juice of bruised stalks, roots, flowers, and fruit—had their uses. It was used alone and in combination with other plants, as today at Pompeii. Scribonius used the juices in making a lozenge to treat intestinal problems (113) and to treat spleen ailments (128). He also used the bramble in medicines for colic (113) and to treat spleen problems in young boys (128, 131). Celsus lists its use in various mixtures, as for dysentery (4.23.2) and for diarrhea (4.26.8).

Soranus lists several uses, including a warm decoction of bramble for skin problems of children (2.52), a decoction of bramble blossoms in sitz baths or injection for hemorrhage of the uterus (3.41), and a decoction of bramble in a sitz bath for gonorrhea (3.46).

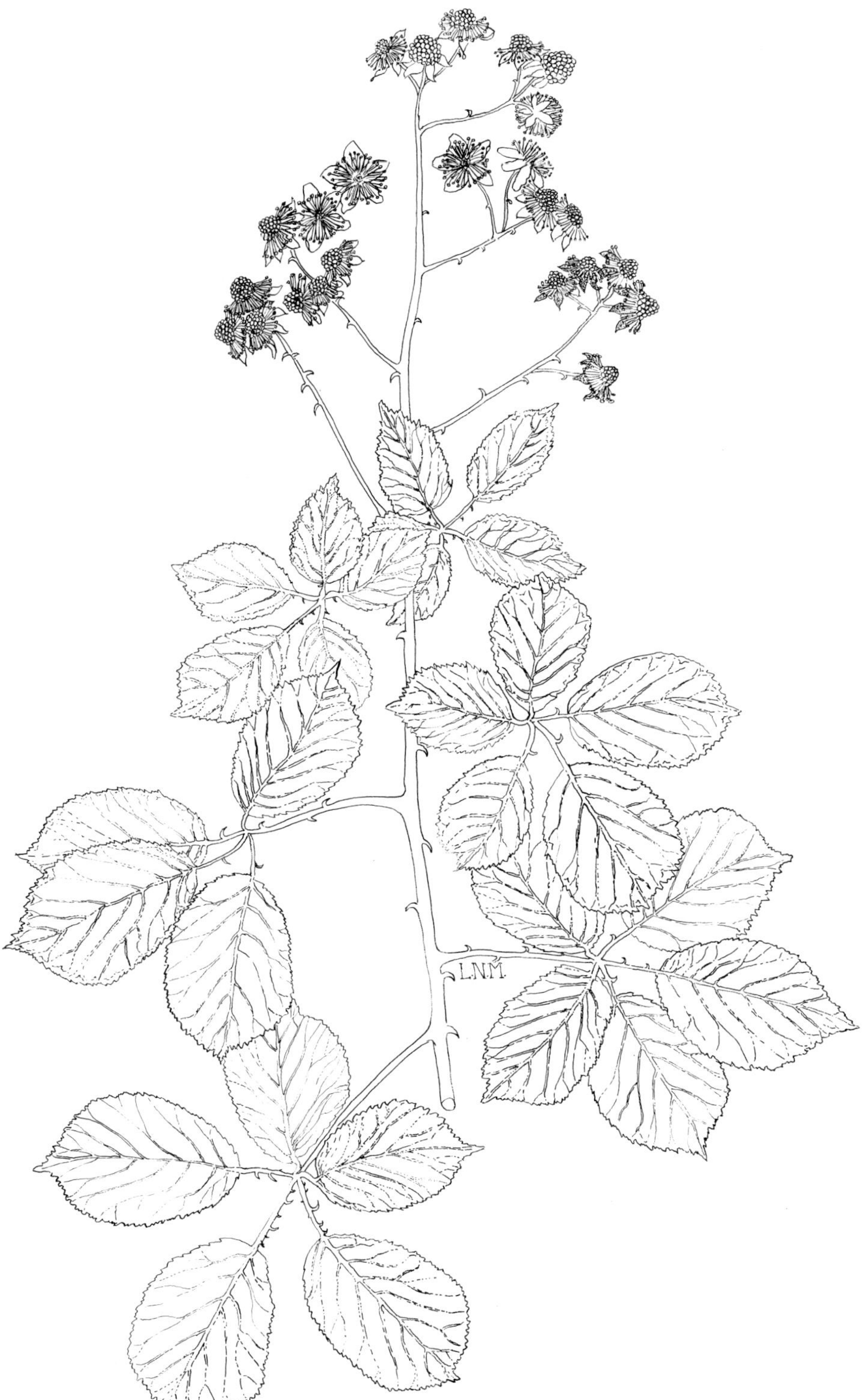
LNM

33 *Ruta graveolens* L.

English, rue

Italian, *ruta*

Rue is a strongly aromatic yellow-flowered subshrub, up to eighty centimeters high. At Pompeii leaves are bruised in warm olive oil to massage aching arms and back. A branch of rue, which has a horrible odor, was put in the swaddling bands in which, until the 1940s, small babies were wrapped from the waist to the feet to keep their legs straight. Since the baby slept with its parents, this discouraged the husband from approaching his wife in the first months after the baby's birth; in other words it served as an antiaphrodisiac. Because its bad odor turns into an agreeable scent if it is put in alcohol, rue is used to give a pleasant aroma to *grappa,* a drink distilled from the dregs of grapes that have been pressed for making wine. After World War II, an infusion of rue leaves in water was used as an abortive in the Pompeii area, as it still is in the vicinity of Rome (Guarrera, p. 143).

Pliny (*HN* 20.131–143) says rue (*ruta*) is "among our chief medicinal plants." He gives a very long list of ailments for which it is a specific, but backache is not one of them. Even though Pliny (*HN* 25.25) says that he is opposed to abortion and does not mention abortives, he gives considerable information, sometimes indirectly, on both birth control and abortion. He says that rue is a plant pregnant women should avoid in their diet for the fetus is killed by it (*HN* 20.143). Soranus gives several prescriptions for abortifacients, one of which includes rue leaves, myrtle, and laurel mixed with wine (1.65). One of his prescriptions for an oral contraceptive includes rue seed (1.63). He adds that this recipe not only prevents conception, but also destroys any already existing. Riddle points out that rue contains pilocarpine, which is given to horses to induce abortion. It is used as an abortifacient among the Hispanic population in New Mexico and Latin America. Laboratory tests on rats have shown its abortifacient and contraceptive effectiveness (Riddle, *Contraception and Abortion,* pp. 28–29). Dioscorides (3.52), in his almost endless list of uses of rue (πήγανον), says it is an emmenagogue, and that wild rue provokes menstruation and expels the fetus. Galen gives a compound prescription for an abortifacient that included rue (*De antidotis* 2.9 = Kühn ed. 14.154).

Celsus gives several medicinal uses of rue as a local irritant. Scribonius uses rue in twelve prescriptions (5, 117, 118, 121, 165, 170, 177, 188, 189, 192, 198, 245), more than he uses any other medicinal plants found at Pompeii.

Pliny says that engravers and painters use it with their food for the sake of their eyes (*HN* 20.134). He reports various uses that Hippocrates made of rue (*HN* 20.139). After Mithridates, king of Pontus, was defeated, the Roman general Pompey found in his cabinet a prescription that would protect against poisoning, written in the king's own handwriting, using twenty rue leaves, two dried walnuts, two figs, and a pinch of salt (*HN* 23.149). Athenaeus, in *The Learned Banquet* (*The Deipnosophists* 3.85.b) reports that the guests of Clearchus, tyrant of Heraclea, ate rue as a preventive, because they knew he wished to poison them.

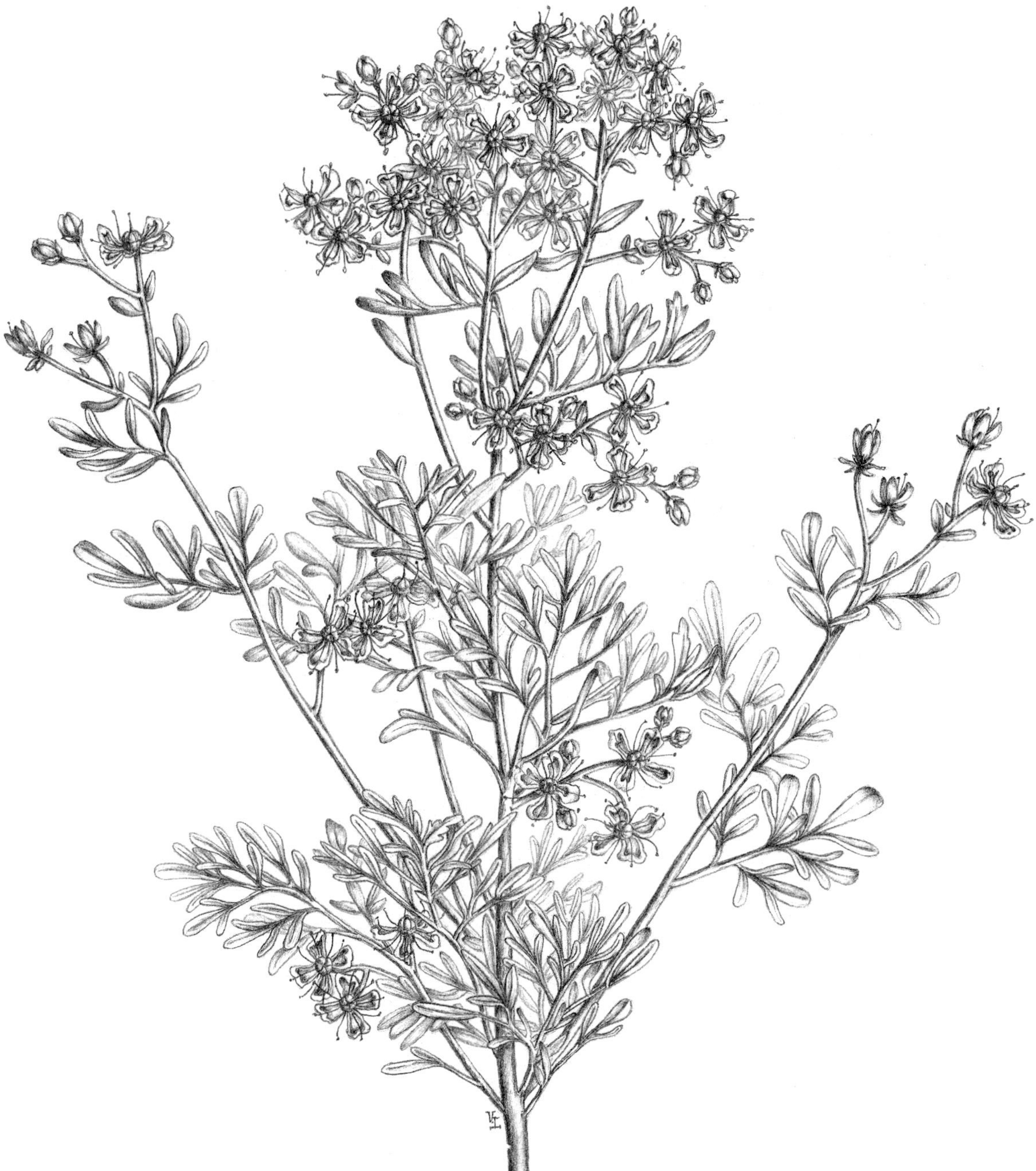

34 *Sambucus nigra* L.

ENGLISH, ELDERBERRY

Italian, *sambuco commune*

The elderberry is a shrub or small tree three to ten meters in height with aromatic cream-white flowers borne in large corymbs (flower clusters) up to twenty centimeters in diameter. The fruit is a round violet-black berry, with red juice. It is found in hedges, woods, and ruins throughout Italy. It flowers in April and May.

The elderberry is a popular medicinal plant throughout Italy today. The flowers are most often used, but all parts of the plant are valued. At Pompeii it is used in an infusion for stomach ailments.

The elderberry has long been known in Europe as a useful plant. Large quantities of the berries have been found in prehistoric sites in Switzerland and north Italy, probably collected for preparing a fermented drink. The Hippocratic Corpus cites its use as a laxative, diuretic, and for gynecological purposes. Pliny (*HN* 24.51–53) gives a large number of medicinal uses for the elderberry (*sambucus, sabucus*). He also says that the berries are used as hair dye. Dioscorides distinguishes between *S. nigra* (ἀκτῆ) (4.174) and *S. ebulus* L. (χαμαιάκτη) (4.175), but he says that they have the same medicinal properties and are used for the same purposes, which is in fact true (Guarrera, p. 38). He describes *S. nigra* as having white flowers and juicy, purplish-black fruit growing in clusters and smacking of wine. Both Pliny and Dioscorides give remedies using all parts of the plant, including the roots, as is the practice in modern Pompeii. Scribonius uses the elderberry in only one prescription, which treats gout (160).

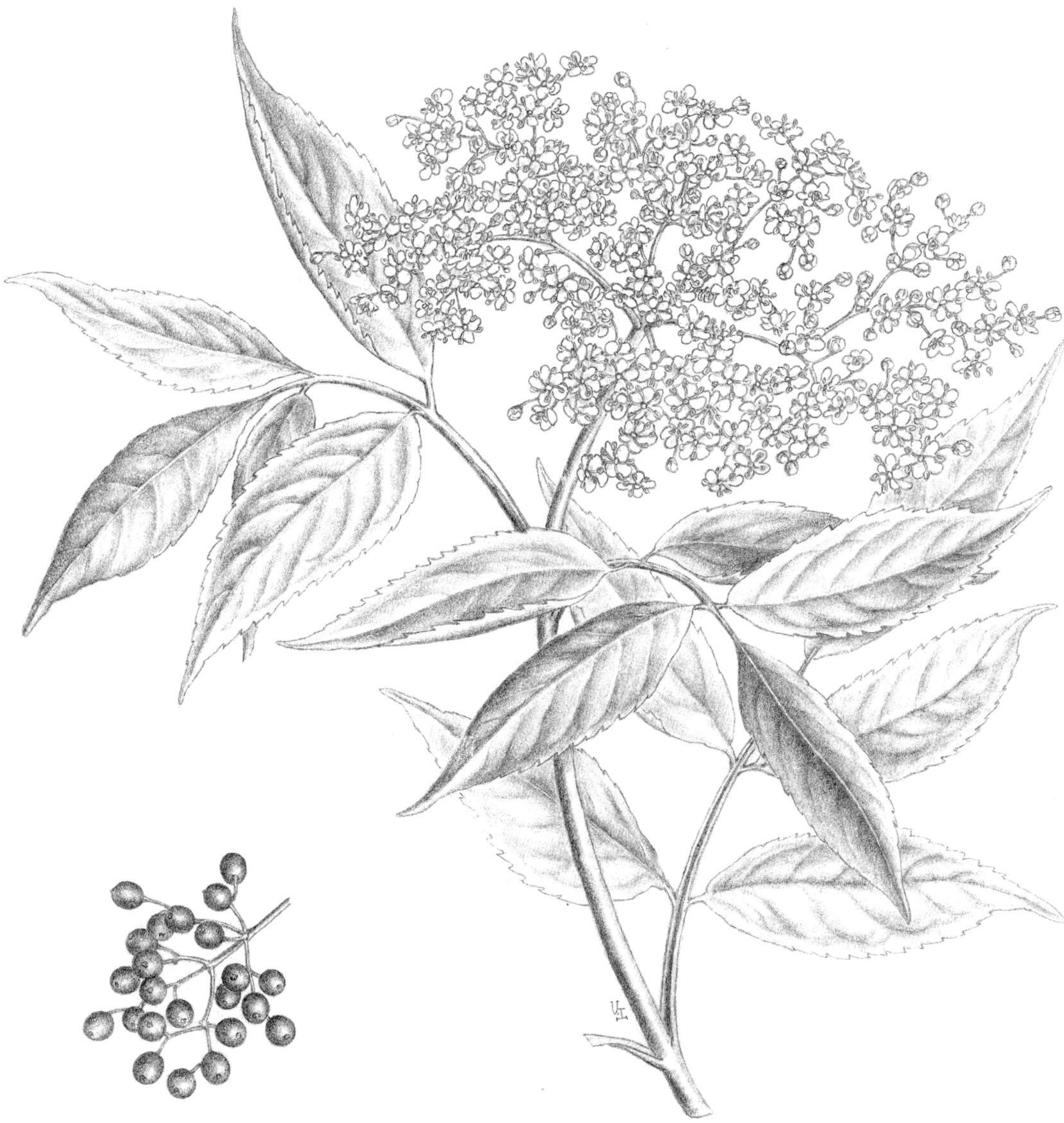

35 *Verbascum sinuatum* L.

English, mullein

Italian, *verbasco*

"Verbascum with the golden flowers" (Pliny *HN* 26.137) grows throughout the excavations at Pompeii and is perhaps the plant most used in this area for medicinal purposes. It was the first medicinal plant that I encountered in my early days at Pompeii. My workmen were digging up these plants to use for curing *fegato* (liver) ailments (see Fig. 1). Mullein is a biennial plant which in the first year produces a basal rosette of leaves (see Fig. 2). It was the root of this plant that the workmen were collecting. The second year the long undulating marginal leaves and tall inflorescences (up to one meter) of yellow flowers appear.

My workmen boiled four mullein roots in water and drank the liquid after meals, one liter per day for six days, as a cure for liver and viscera problems. They said that an infusion also cured jaundice. For fever caused by intestinal ailments, the roots are washed well, boiled in water, the liquid filtered in a cloth, and one glass of the liquid drunk as often as needed.

Later I met an old man, who had worked in the excavations for forty-two years, as he was collecting medicinal plants—mullein and vervain. He had six small mullein plants, which he said he would boil for twenty minutes in one to two liters of water, and then drink one liter of the liquid per day, before or after meals. He, too, said it would completely cure *fegato* ailments.

In antiquity mullein root was also used for looseness of the bowels (Pliny *HN* 26.44), but it was a specific for many other ills. Pliny (*HN* 25.120) says there were several kinds of mullein (*verbascum*). However, they all have the same properties. He gives a long list of the medicinal uses of *verbascum*. He claims that its potency is so great that even beasts of burden that are not only suffering from cough but also broken-winded are relieved by a draught (*HN* 25.29). For coughs, and pains in the side and in the chest, mullein with rue is taken in water (*HN* 26.31).

Dioscorides describes various kinds of mullein under the Greek name *phlomos* (φλόμος), giving their many medicinal uses, adding that the golden-colored flowers dye the hair (4.104).

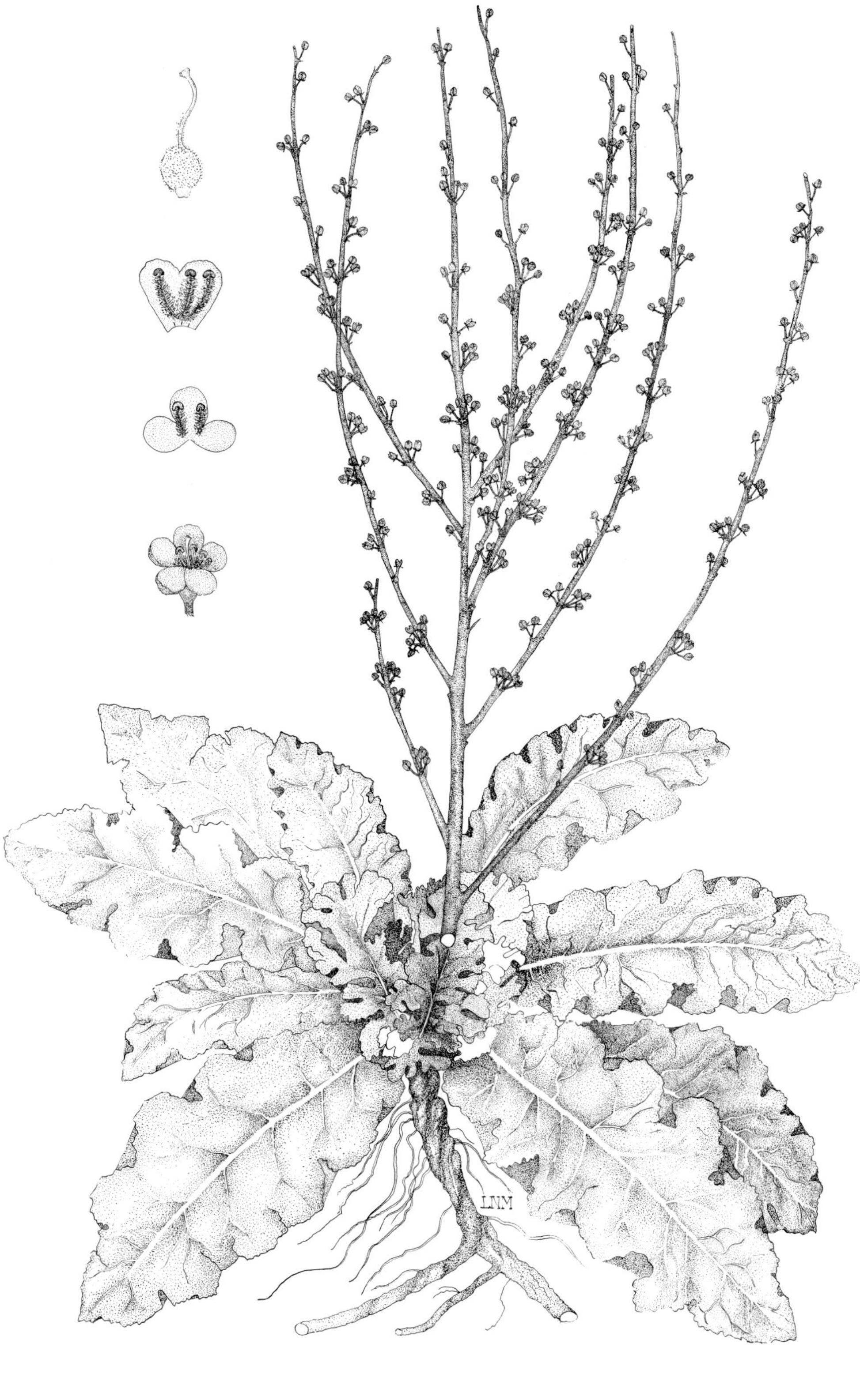
LNM

36 *Verbena officinalis* L.

English, vervain, verbena

Italian, *verbena, erba colombina, erba crocina*

This hairy perennial, up to sixty centimeters or more in height, with deeply cut leaves and long, narrow spikes of tiny lilac flowers, grows in waste places around the entire Mediterranean. Its pollen was identified in the core taken at Lake Avernus.

Vervain is one of the medicinal plants most used at Pompeii today. An infusion of vervain is a specific for liver ailments and also used to purify the urine. The gardener in the House of Pansa recommended drinking two glasses of water a day in which vervain had been boiled, one in the morning and the other in the evening. Another workman insisted that eight plants should be boiled in water for one-half hour, and a liter drunk after meals! The old man whom I met collecting mullein and vervain (see above, no. 35) said that similar amounts of verbena could be used in the same way to cure *fegato* ailments. He said *verbena* was the best of all medicinal plants—it would cure all maladies. *Verbena* and mullein were the only two medicinal plants that he used. The women who lived in the excavations also stressed the importance of vervain for liver problems; they boil two branches in one liter of water for fifteen minutes and recommend one glass of the cold liquid a day.

Hippocrates is said to have considered vervain to be one of the few cure-all herbs. Pliny gives an almost endless list of the medicinal uses of vervain (*verbenaca*), which botanists agree is *Verbena officinalis* L. He says that it is a cure for troubles of all the internal organs (*HN* 26.37,38). If a dining-couch is sprinkled with water in which this plant has been soaked, the entertainment becomes merrier (*HN* 25.107). Scribonius has only three prescriptions that contain vervain (142, 205, 232).

Dioscorides (4.60) also refers to vervain (περιστερεών) as the sacred plant. He describes it in greater detail: it is a cubit (forty-six centimeters) or more in height and has deeply cut leaves and thin purple flowers. He gives many of the same medicinal uses that Pliny does. Dioscorides said that it was called *peristereōn* (from the Greek word for "dove"), because the doves liked to stay around it. It is interesting that one of the common names for this plant in Italy today is *colombina,* "little dove."

This plant held a place of honor among the ancient Greeks and Romans completely inconsistent with its humble appearance. It was extremely important in ancient Roman political and religious life. Pliny says that no plant was so renowned among the Romans as the sacred plant which the Latin writers call *verbenaca.* It was carried to the enemy by envoys when a declaration of war was made. With it the table of Jupiter was swept on his feast days, and homes cleansed and purified (*HN* 25.105).

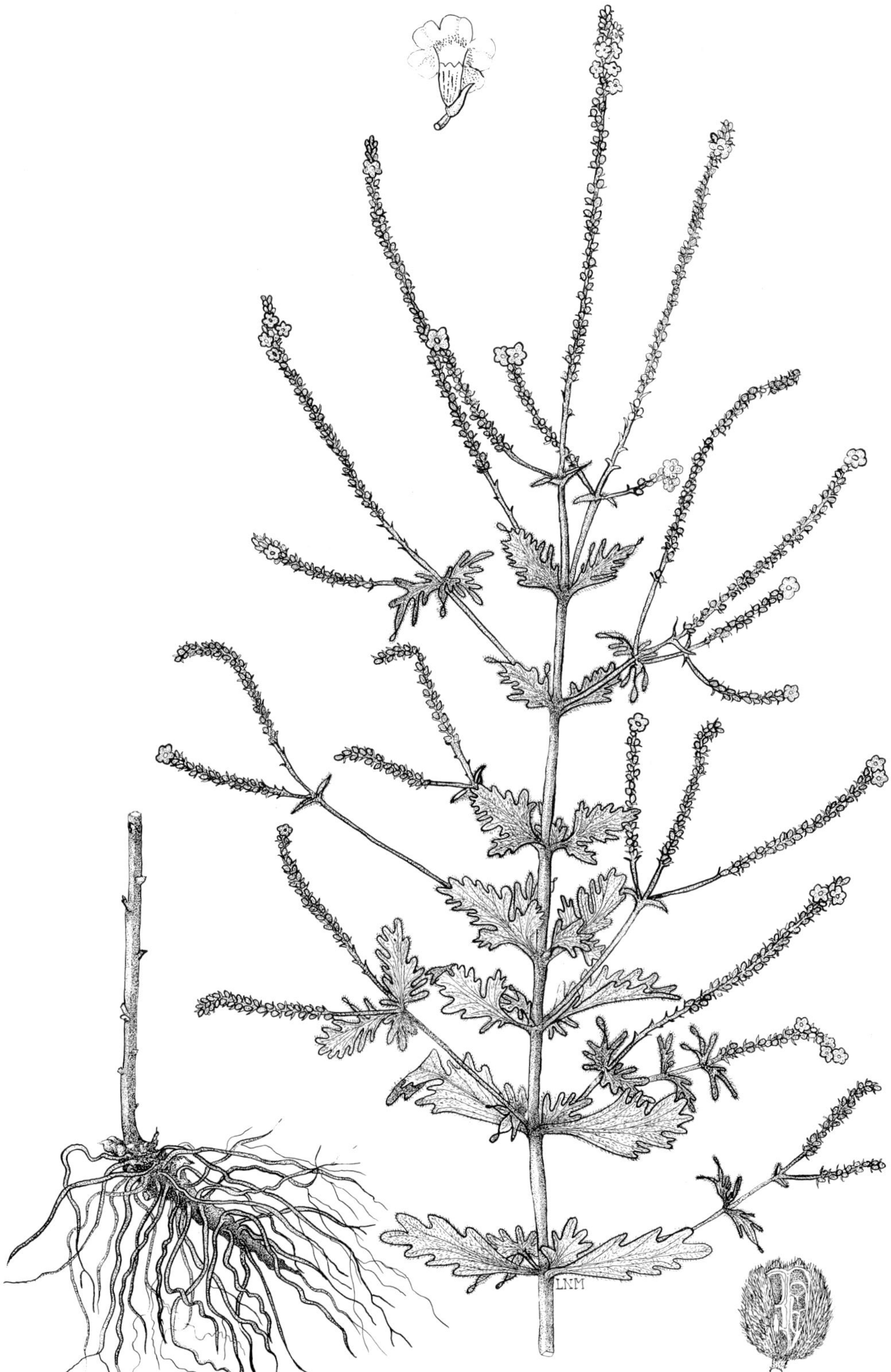
LNM

Ancient Authors Cited or Quoted

Apicius. *The Roman Cookery Book.* Translated by Barbara Flower and Elisabeth Rosenbaum. London and New York, 1960.

Apuleius Platonicus. *Herbarium.* (See *Herbarium Apulei* published by Joannes Philippus de Lignamine, Rome, 1481; facsimile Milan, 1979.)

Athenaeus. *The Deipnosophists.* Loeb Classical Library (hereafter LCL). 7 vols. Translated by C. B. Gulick. London, 1963–1970.

Aurelius Victor. *Epitome de Caesaribus.* Rome, 1696.

Cato. *De re rustica.* LCL. Translated by W. D. Hooper, revised by H. B. Ash. Cambridge, Mass., and London, 1954.

Celsus. *De medicina.* LCL. 3 vols. Translated by W. G. Spencer. Cambridge, Mass., and London, 1938.

Cicero. *Pro Murena.* Translated by C. Macdonald in LCL *Rhetorical Treatises,* vol. 10. Cambridge, Mass., and London, 1976.

Codex Vindobonensis Medicus Graecus. 5 vols. (full-color facsimile of the Juliana Anicia Codex). Graz, 1965–1970.

Columella. *De re rustica.* LCL. 3 vols. Vol. 1 translated by H. B. Ash, Cambridge, Mass., and London, 1960. Vols. 2 and 3 translated by E. S. Forster and E. H. Heffner. Vol. 2, Cambridge, Mass., and London, 1968. Vol. 3, Cambridge, Mass., and London, 1955.

Dioscorides. *De materia medica libri quinque.* Edited by Max Wellman. 3 vols. Berlin, 1906–1914; reprinted 1958. (The best text; no translation.)

———. *The Greek Herbal of Dioscorides.* Edited by Robert T. Gunther. New York, 1934; reprinted 1968.

Galen. *De alimentorum facultatibus* and *De ptisana.* In *Corpus Medicorum Graecorum* (the best text) 5.4.2. Edited by K. Koch, G. Helmreich, C. Kalbfleisch, and O. Hartlich. Leipzig and Berlin, 1923.

———. *Opera.* Edited by Karl G. Kühn. 22 vols. Hildesheim, 1821–1833; reprinted 1964–1965. Works cited: *Commentarii I in Hippocratis librum de humoribus; De alimentarum facultatibus; De antidotis; De locis affectis: De ptisana; De simplicium medicamentorum temperamentis ac facultatibus.*

Hippocrates. LCL. 8 vols. Translated by W. H. G. Jones. Cambridge, Mass., 1923–1931.

Horace. *Satires.* LCL. Translated by H. R. Fairclough. London and New York, 1926.

Juvenal. LCL. Translated by G. G. Ramsey. Rev. ed. Cambridge, Mass., and London, 1957.

Martial. *Epigrams.* LCL. 3 vols. Translated by W. C. A. Ker. New York and London, 1919–1920.

Ovid. *Fasti.* LCL. Translated by J. G. Frazer. New York and London, 1931.

———. *Metamorphoses.* LCL. 2 vols. Translated by F. J. Miller. Vol. 1, Cambridge, Mass., 1976. Vol. 2, Cambridge, Mass., 1977.

Pausanius. *Description of Greece.* LCL. 5 vols. Translated by W. H. Jones and H. A. Omerod. Cambridge, Mass., 1918–1935.

Pliny the Elder. *Natural History.* LCL. Vols. 4, 5 translated by H. Rackham, Cambridge, Mass., and London, 1960, 1961. Vols. 6, 7 translated by W. H. S. Jones, Cambridge, Mass., and London, 1951, 1956.

Pliny the Younger. *Letters and Panegyricus.* LCL. 2 vols. Translated by Betty Radice. Cambridge, Mass., and London, 1969.

Plutarch. *The Parallel Lives.* LCL. Vol. 3. Translated by B. Perrin. Cambridge, Mass., and London, 1916; reprinted 1951.

Scribonius Largus. *Compositiones.* Teubner. Edited by S. Sconocchia. Leipzig, 1983.

Soranus. *Gynecology.* Edited and translated by Oswei Temkin. Baltimore, 1956.

Strabo. *Geography.* LCL. 8 vols. Translated by H. L. Jones. New York and London, 1931–1949.

Theocritus [included in] *Greek Bucolic Poets.* LCL. Translated by J. M. Edwards. New York and London, 1950.

Theophrastus. *Enquiry into Plants.* LCL. 2 vols. Translated by Sir Arthur Hort. New York and London. Vol. 1 reprinted 1968. Vol. 2 reprinted 1961.

Tibullus. LCL. Translated by F. W. Comish. New York and London, 1912.

Virgil. *Eclogues, Georgics, Aeneid and Minor Poems.* LCL. 2 vols. Translated by H. Rushton Fairclough. New York and London, 1922.

Select Bibliography of Secondary Sources

Guarrera, P. M. *Il patrimonio etnobotanico del Lazio.* Rome, 1994.

Hepper, F. N. *Pharaoh's Flowers.* London, 1990.

Hopkins, Keith. "Contraception in the Roman Empire." *Comparative Studies in Society and History* 8 (1965–1966): 124–151.

Jashemski, Wilhelmina F. *The Gardens of Pompeii, Herculaneum, and the Villas Destroyed by Vesuvius.* Vol. 1, New Rochelle, N.Y., 1979. Vol. 2, New Rochelle, N.Y., 1993.

Jashemski, Wilhelmina F., and Frederick G. Meyer, eds. *The Natural History of Pompeii and the Other Vesuvian Sites.* Forthcoming.

Köhler, Eugen. *Medizinal-Pflanzen.* Edited by G. Pabst. 3 vols. Gera, 1887–1889; reprinted 1990–1991.

Lindsell, Alice. "Was Theocritus a Botanist?" *Greece and Rome* 6: 17 (1937): 78–93.

Mau, August. *Pompeii: Its Life and Art.* Translated by Francis W. Kelsey. 2nd ed. New York, 1902; reprinted, New Rochelle, N.Y., 1982.

Meyer, Frederick G. "Food Plants Identified from Carbonized Remains at Pompeii and Other Vesuvian Sites." In *Studia Pompeiana and Classica,* vol. 1, edited by Robert I. Curtis. New Rochelle, N.Y., 1988.

Ricciardi, Massimo, and Giuseppa Grazia Aprile. "Identification of Some Carbonized Plant Remains from the Archaeological Area of Oplontis." In *Studia Pompeiana and Classica,* vol. 1, edited by Robert I. Curtis. New Rochelle, N.Y., 1988.

Ricciardi, Massimo, Giuseppa Grazia Aprile, Vincenzo La Valva, and Giuseppe Caputo. "La flora del Somma-Vesuvio." Extract from *Bollettino della Società dei Naturalisti in Napoli* 95 (1986): 3–121.

Riddle, John M. *Contraception and Abortion from the Ancient World to the Renaissance.* Cambridge, Mass., and London, 1992.

———. *Dioscorides on Pharmacy and Medicine.* Austin, 1985.

Saccardo, P. A. *Cronologia della flora italiana.* Padua, 1909; reprinted, Bologna, 1971.

Singer, Charles. "The Herbal in Antiquity and Its Transition to Later Ages." *Journal of Hellenistic Studies* 47 (1927): 1–52.

Stannard, Jerry. "Pliny and Roman Botany." *Isis* 56.4: 186 (1965): 420–425.

Tolkowsky, S. *Hesperides: A History of the Culture and Use of Citrus Fruits.* London, 1983.

Zangheri, Pietro. *Flora Italica.* 2 vols. Padua. 1976.

List of Illustrations

Chapter 1: Figures

Chapter II: Plant Portraits

1. *Adiantum capillus-veneris* L. Illustrator: Lillian Nicholson Meyer and Victoria I.
2. *Alcea rosea* L. Illustrator: Victoria I after Köhler.
3. *Artemisia absinthium* L. Illustrator: Lillian Nicholson Meyer after N. Robert.
4. *Calamintha nepeta* (L.) Savi. Illustrator: Victoria I.
5. *Castanea sativa* Miller. Illustrator: Victoria I.
6. *Centranthus ruber* (L.) DC. Illustrator: Victoria I.
7. *Chamomilla recutita* (L.) Rauschert. Illustrator: Lillian Nicholson Meyer.
8. *Cichorium intybus* L. Illustrator: Lillian Nicholson Meyer.
9. *Citrus limon* (L.) Burm. f. Illustrator: Victoria I after Köhler.
10. *Cyclamen hederifolium* Aiton. Illustrator: Lillian Nicholson Meyer.
11. *Cynodon dactylon* (L.) Pers. Illustrator: Victoria I.
12. *Delphinium halteratum* Sibth. & Sm. Illustrator: Victoria I.
13. *Diplotaxis tenuifolia* (L.) DC. Illustrator: Victoria I.
14. *Eucalyptus camaldulensis* Dehnh. Illustrator: Victoria I.
15. *Ficus carica* L. Illustrator: Victoria I.
16. *Foeniculum vulgare* Miller. Illustrator: Victoria I.
17. *Hordeum vulgare* L. Illustrator: Victoria I.
18. *Hypericum perforatum* L. Illustrator: Lillian Nicholson Meyer after Chastillon.
19. *Juglans regia* L. Illustrator: Lillian Nicholson Meyer.
20. *Lactuca sativa* L. Illustrator: Victoria I.
21. *Laurus nobilis* L. Illustrator: Lillian Nicholson Meyer.
22. *Lobularia maritima* (L.) Desv. Illustrator: Victoria I.
23. *Malus domestica* Borkh. Illustrator: Victoria I after Köhler.
24. *Malva sylvestris* L. Illustrator: Lillian Nicholson Meyer.
25. *Mentha suaveolens* Ehrh. Illustrator: Victoria I.
26. *Myrtus communis* L. Illustrator: Victoria I.
27. *Parietaria officinalis* L. Illustrator: Lillian Nicholson Meyer.
28. *Petroselinum crispum* (Miller) A. W. Hill. Illustrator: Victoria I after Köhler.
29. *Plantago major* L. Illustrator: Lillian Nicholson Meyer.
30. *Polygonum aviculare* L. Illustrator: Lillian Nicholson Meyer.
31. *Portulaca oleracea* L. Illustrator: Victoria I after L. Fuchs.
32. *Rubus ulmifolius* Schott. Illustrator: Lillian Nicholson Meyer.
33. *Ruta graveolens* L. Illustrator: Lillian Nicholson Meyer and Victoria I.
34. *Sambucus nigra* L. Illustrator: Victoria I after Köhler.
35. *Verbascum sinuatum* L. Illustrator: Lillian Nicholson Meyer.
36. *Verbena officinalis* L. Illustrator: Lillian Nicholson Meyer.

Index

Numbers in italics refer to page numbers of illustrations.

Greek Index